Updates in Surgery

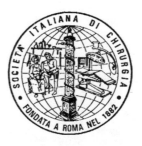

Giampiero Campanelli
Editor

Inguinal Hernia Surgery

Foreword by
Francesco Corcione

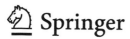 Springer

Editor
Giampiero Campanelli
University of Insubria
General and Day Surgery Unit
Center of Research and High Specialization for the Pathologies of Abdominal Wall
and Surgical Treatment and Repair of Abdominal Hernia
Istituto Clinico Sant'Ambrogio
Milan, Italy
President, The European Hernia Society

The publication and the distribution of this volume have been supported by the Italian Society of Surgery

ISSN 2280-9848   ISSN 2281-0854 (electronic)
Updates in Surgery
ISBN 978-88-470-3970-4   ISBN 978-88-470-3947-6 (eBook)

DOI 10.1007/978-88-470-3947-6

Cover design: eStudio Calamar S.L.
External publishing product development: Scienzaperta, Novate Milanese (Milan), Italy
Typesetting: Graphostudio, Milan, Italy

This Springer imprint is published by Springer Nature
Springer-Verlag Italia S.r.l. – Via Decembrio 28 – I-20137 Milan
Springer is a part of Springer Science+Business Media (www.springer.com)

Foreword

The famous statement of Edoardo Bassini still appears very relevant. Is it useful to talk about hernia today? Is it useful to dedicate to hernia repair, a so-called minor surgery, a biennial report at SIC? In my opinion the answer is "yes, it is necessary". Hernia is not a minor pathology. It requires a deep knowledge of surgical anatomy and a high level of surgical skill to master all the different existing procedures.

I believe that very few topics have attracted as much attention as the treatment of hernia over the last 25 years. Twenty-five years ago hernia repair required a middle-to-long hospital stay (8-10 days) and had a high rate of recurrences. Moreover, only two or three standardized procedures were available and very few companies were interested in investing money in this field. Today, hernia is treated on an outpatient basis, the recurrence rate is very low, and surgeons can choose from dozens of procedures and more or less new materials and devices that reach the market every day.

New problems have emerged as well, such as recurrence after hernia repair with mesh, prosthesis infection and rejection, postoperative neuralgia and other conditions. These are only a few of the downsides that this revolution has brought, which has resulted in many surgeons dedicating themselves to the study and treatment of hernia.

Prof. Giampiero Campanelli is one of these surgeons. He has dedicated himself to this condition since he was young and he has acquired the experience, skill and knowledge of surgical anatomy that put him in the limelight of many national and international surgical societies to the point that he became President of the European Hernia Society.

In this context, I believe Prof. Campanelli is undoubtedly the best suited to deal with such a delicate and complex issue. I would like to thank Prof. Campanelli and his expert collaborators for the contribution delivered to this congress.

I would also like to thank Springer, as always and more than ever, for their organizational effectiveness and editorial expertise in assisting in all the reports of Italian Society of Surgery.

Rome, September 2016   Francesco Corcione
President, Italian Society of Surgery

Preface

Our clinical experience, mainly focused on the study and surgical repair of abdominal wall defects (from the simplest to the most complex, from the most common to the rarest), started in the first half of the 80s, even before the introduction of modern prosthetic materials.

In the following years, with the advent of implants (meshes and plugs), many new surgical techniques were proposed and tested worldwide for the treatment of abdominal hernias, some of them performed with traditional laparotomy, others with laparoscopy or even with robotic surgery, reflecting the technological advances which we have witnessed in the last 30 years.

During all these years we made ourselves global promoters of this amazing surgical discipline, one that today fully deserves to be defined as highly specialized, a nascent art that requires great professional and intellectual dedication to be understood in its vastness and depth.

This exciting scientific endeavor led us soon to consider, among other aspects, that we cannot limit ourselves to adopting one standardized operating procedure for all patients with the same type of hernia, but, on the contrary, we must distinguish the different indications and most appropriate treatment options for each individual case and for each single patient.

For these reasons we like to define this surgery as a "tailored surgery".

Of course, in the "international" light of the guidelines that we have contributed to realize in these years we can state, without doubt, that for the routine repair of daily primary uncomplicated inguinal hernias, a perfect knowledge of at least the Liechtenstein technique and TAPP repair is enough for the majority of general non-specialized surgeons.

Indeed, every intervention we propose must be as far as possible adapted to the individual patient; in particular, we have to consider the patient's constitution, the presence of possible comorbidities, the patient's age, gender, overall physical performance, and personal daily needs and, of course, the quality of the tissues involved, the anatomy and the type of hernia defect, which must be properly identified and characterized, and, finally, the possible improvement in quality of life achievable in each single case.

All these parameters are reflected on the most appropriate choice not only of prosthetic material but also of surgical approach. The prosthetic material is selected from among a large variety of materials that may or may not be used (synthetic or biological, soft or rigid, with different elastic-physical, morphological and structural characteristics), and must be suitably shaped and calibrated in relation to the existing anatomical differences between individuals, considering the pathophysiological dynamics involved in the genesis of the disease, and the total and actual size of the hernia defect identified in each case. Similarly, the best surgical approach is chosen based on the above parameters and the additional purposes to be achieved with a given type of repair.

No doubt the first among these additional purposes is the respect of the physiology of the abdominal wall, which must always be preserved to the greatest possible extent, by respecting and protecting the noble structures and sparing the nerves of the region involved in the repair, so as to minimize postoperative pain and ensure patient comfort with a more rapid and efficient recovery of the patient's usual daily activities.

Even the mastery of surgical techniques to be performed under local anesthesia, which allow patients to return home within hours of the surgery, plays an important role in this concept of "tailored surgery".

To give a few examples, in surgery of primary unilateral groin hernia, we generally choose to perform sutureless and tension-free techniques with a mini-incision (2.5 to 6 cm), which guarantee a very low recurrence rate in the long term (0.02%), comparable to the rates observed for the widespread Lichtenstein's technique (which today still represents the golden standard treatment for this type of pathology, together with the laparoscopic TAPP approach). These techniques significantly reduce suture-related postoperative pain and can be easily performed under local anesthesia on a day-case basis.

We have personally led and developed many scientific studies also concerning fixation of the different types of meshes with fibrin glue, which shows excellent results in terms of efficacy and tolerability, as an alternative to traditional sutures. These devices are particularly suitable for the treatment of the hernias in the young and in athletes.

Nevertheless, in each case we have achieved great accuracy in detecting whether such techniques are suitable and fruitful for the individual patient: in other words, we have the option of using other kinds of repair such as the preperitoneal approach, anterior or posterior, plug, with absorbable (biologic) meshes, dynamic repair and, of course, laparoscopy. The laparoscopic approach can, for instance, be useful for the repair of bilateral groin hernia, whether primary or recurrent. Laparoscopy can be the first choice for incisional hernia repair in obese patients, in athletes with a small ventral defect, or in those patients who have already undergone a previous laparotomic repair.

Even in the open surgery of "simple" incisional hernias it is possible to adopt sutureless and tension-free techniques, exploiting the law of Pascal and employing fibrin glue for fixing the mesh in most of the cases.

In the presence, for example, of a real loss of substance, it is appropriate to fill the gap with an at least partially biologic prosthesis, which remains in contact with the viscera without causing adhesions and other well-known complications. In the same cases, the knowledge of and the ability to perform each kind of component separation (open, laparoscopic, anterior, posterior transversus abdominis release) is mandatory in order to really be able to realize an appropriate tailored approach.

The extent of the repair must be carefully evaluated in the preoperative phase, whatever the surgical technique that will be proposed to the patient, with careful choice of the most appropriate prosthetic materials: also the most suitable size of mesh must be well thought out and commensurate to the type of hernia defect identified in each case.

This eclectic approach requires, on the one hand, deep knowledge, culture and skill in all the possible techniques and, on the other, a continuous exchange of information among peers to enable a real and honest evaluation of results and ensure the best possible outcome for patients.

Milan, September 2016   Giampiero Campanelli
                                                        President, The European Hernia Society

Contents

All web addresses have been checked and were correct at time of printing.

Contributors

Fabio Amatucci CERGAS, Centre for Research on Health and Social Care Management, Università Bocconi, Milan, Italy

Parviz K. Amid Lichtenstein-Amid Hernia Clinic, David Geffen School of Medicine at the University of California, Los Angeles, Santa Monica, California, USA

Kristoffer Andresen Department of Surgery, Herlev Hospital, Herlev, Denmark

Rafael Azuaje Hernia Institute of Florida, Miami, Florida, USA

Conrad D. Ballecer Center for Minimally Invasive and Robotic Surgery, Peoria, Arizona, USA

Frederik Christiaan Berrevoet Department of General and Hepatopancreaticobiliairy Surgery and Liver Transplantation, Ghent University Hospital, Ghent, Belgium

Waqar Bhatti Hip and Groin Clinic, Spire Manchester Hospital, Manchester, United Kingdom

Piero Giovanni Bruni General and Day Surgery Unit, Center of Research and High Specialization for the Pathologies of Abdominal Wall and Surgical Treatment and Repair of Abdominal Hernia, Istituto Clinico Sant'Ambrogio, Milan, Italy

Giampiero Campanelli University of Insubria, General and Day Surgery Unit, Center of Research and High Specialization for the Pathologies of Abdominal Wall and Surgical Treatment and Repair of Abdominal Hernia, Istituto Clinico Sant'Ambrogio, Milan, Italy

Marta Cavalli General and Day Surgery Unit, Center of Research and High Specialization for the Pathologies of Abdominal Wall and Surgical Treatment and Repair of Abdominal Hernia, Istituto Clinico Sant'Ambrogio, Milan, Italy

David C. Chen Lichtenstein-Amid Hernia Clinic, David Geffen School of Medicine at the University of California, Los Angeles, Santa Monica, California, USA

Max Fehily Hip and Groin Clinic, Spire Manchester Hospital, Manchester, United Kingdom

Edward L. Felix Marian Regional Medical Center, Santa Maria, California, USA

René H. Fortelny Department of General, Visceral and Oncological Surgery, Wilhelminen Spital, Vienna, Austria

Arthur I. Gilbert Miller-Miami Medical School, Hernia Institute of Florida, Miami, Florida, USA

Dalila Patrizia Greco Day and Week Surgery Unit, Multi Specialist Surgery Department, ASST Grande Ospedale Metropolitano Niguarda, Milan, Italy

Ivy N. Haskins Cleveland Clinic Comprehensive Hernia Center, Cleveland Clinic Foundation, Cleveland, Ohio, USA

Saurabh Jamdar Department of General and Hernia Surgery, Central Manchester Foundation Trust, Manchester Royal Infirmary, Manchester, United Kingdom

David Jones Hip and Groin Clinic, Spire Manchester Hospital, Manchester, United Kingdom

Doug Jones Hip and Groin Clinic, Spire Manchester Hospital, Manchester, United Kingdom

Giel G. Koning Department of Surgery, Division of Vascular and Transplant Surgery, Radboud University Medical Center, Nijmegen, The Netherlands

Jan F. Kukleta Visceral Surgery Unit, Hirslanden Klinik Im Park, Zurich, Switzerland

Karl A. LeBlanc Surgeons Group of Baton Rouge, Our Lady of the Lake Physician Group, Baton Rouge, Louisiana, USA

Davide Lomanto Minimally Invasive Surgical Centre, Department of Surgery, YLL School of Medicine, National University of Singapore, Singapore

Andrea Morlacchi General and Day Surgery Unit, Center of Research and High Specialization for the Pathologies of Abdominal Wall and Surgical Treatment and Repair of Abdominal Hernia, Istituto Clinico Sant'Ambrogio, Milan, Italy

John W. Murphy William Beaumont Hospital-Troy, Bloomfield Hills, Michigan, USA

Philippe Ngo The Hernia Institute Paris, Paris, France

David K. Nguyen Department of Surgery, David Geffen School of Medicine at the University of California, Los Angeles, Santa Monica, California, USA

Giovanni Andrea Padula CERGAS, Centre for Research on Health and Social Care Management, Università Bocconi, Milan, Italy

Edouard P. Pélissier The Hernia Institute Paris, Paris, France

Alexander H. Petter-Puchner Department of General, Visceral and Oncological Surgery, Wilhelminen Spital, Vienna, Austria

Brian E. Prebil Center for Minimally Invasive and Robotic Surgery, Peoria, Arizona, USA

Michael J. Rosen Cleveland Clinic Comprehensive Hernia Center, Cleveland Clinic Foundation, Cleveland, Ohio, USA

Jacob Rosenberg Department of Surgery, Herlev Hospital, Herlev, Denmark

Aali J. Sheen Department of General and Hernia Surgery, Central Manchester Foundation Trust, Manchester Royal Infirmary, Manchester, United Kingdom

Marc Soler Centre de Chirurgie Pariétale, Cagnes sur Mer, France

Eva Lourdes Sta. Clara Minimally Invasive Surgical Centre, Department of Surgery, YLL School of Medicine, National University of Singapore, Singapore

Shirin Towfigh Beverly Hills Hernia Center, Beverly Hills, Cedars-Sinai Medical Center, Department of Surgery, California, USA

Jerrold Young Miller-Miami Medical School, Hernia Institute of Florida, Miami, Florida, USA

Lichtenstein Tension-free Hernioplasty

David K. Nguyen, Parviz K. Amid, and David C. Chen

1.1 Introduction

The inguinal hernia has plagued humankind since the advent of recorded history. Edoardo Bassini's seminal presentation to the Italian Surgical Society in 1887 of a durable native tissue-based technique for restoring the integrity of the inguinal floor ushered in a new era of hernia surgery based upon understanding of the anatomy and mechanics of the inguinal canal. Since then, numerous tissue repairs of the inguinal canal have been described in the surgical literature and were considered the gold standard until the 1980s.

Weak abdominal wall tissue was recognized as an intrinsic cause of inguinal hernias even in the 19th century. However, early attempts at recreating the tensile strength of fascia and tendon with prosthetic materials were plagued by rejection and infection. In 1959, Usher introduced polypropylene mesh – a strong, lightweight, flexible, and biologically inert material. Scientific advancements broadened the understanding of hernia formation as a metabolic process not solely caused by mechanical forces. Alterations to collagen type I to type III ratios and an imbalance of protease and antiprotease lead to impaired hydroxylation of proline. These changes are associated with a weakening of the fibro-connective tissues of the groin, leading to the development of inguinal hernias. The availability of suitable prosthetic materials and the contradictory nature of placing defective, weakened inguinal tissue under tension renewed interest in prosthetic-based, tension-free groin hernia repairs.

In 1984, Irving Lichtenstein, Alex Schulman, and Parviz Amid of the Lichtenstein Hernia Institute in Los Angeles began a protocol-based study to routinely use prosthetic mesh for inguinal hernia repair. The Lichtenstein tension-free hernioplasty is a result of their efforts to circumvent the degenerative nature of the groin hernia and the detrimental effects of suture line tension. Rather than placing

D.C. Chen (✉)
Lichtenstein-Amid Hernia Clinic, David Geffen School of Medicine at the University of California, Los Angeles
Santa Monica, California, USA
e-mail: dcchen@ucla.edu

G. Campanelli (Ed), *Inguinal Hernia Surgery*,
Updates in Surgery
DOI: 10.1007/978-88-470-3947-6_1, © Springer-Verlag Italia 2017

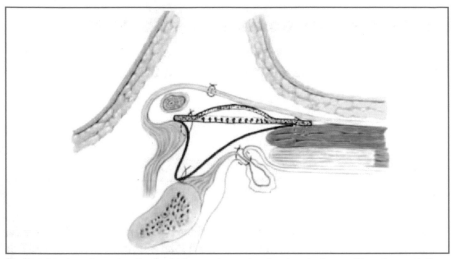

Fig. 1.1 Ideal configuration for the Lichtenstein tension-free hernioplasty with an inverted direct hernia sac. Sagittal view. The *black dotted line* is not recommended due to tension. The *solid black line* shows the position of a femoral hernia repair

defective tissues under tension by apposing them with suture, mesh is used to reinforce the entire inguinal floor. It is situated between the transversalis fascia that forms the inguinal floor and the external oblique aponeurosis. It extends from the internal ring to well beyond Hesselbach's triangle, providing adequate mesh-tissue interface. Upon increased intra-abdominal pressures associated with straining, the external oblique aponeurosis contracts and applies counter-pressure on the mesh, thus making intra-abdominal pressures favorable to the repair [1]. With a tissue-based repair, these same mechanics place added tension on the suture line predisposing it to failure and recurrence. Mesh positioned in this location provides a repair that is both therapeutic and prophylactic (Fig. 1.1) addressing the current herniation as well as protecting the inguinal floor from future metabolic and mechanical disturbances.

1.1.1   Preoperative Evaluation

The risk of complications from an inguinal hernia repair is low. Surgery to repair an inguinal hernia or its complications may leave the patient at risk for infection, bleeding, recurrence, pain, visceral or vascular injury, spermatic cord injury, testicular atrophy or loss, hematoma or seroma formation, nerve entrapment, urinary retention, bladder injury, osteitis pubis, or intra-abdominal adhesions. Most of these are very low risk events. Rates of recurrence, a notable morbidity, vary with ranges from 1 to 7% for indirect and from 4 to 10% for direct hernias [2–5]. The incidence of postherniorrhaphy pain is variable from 0.5 to over 60%

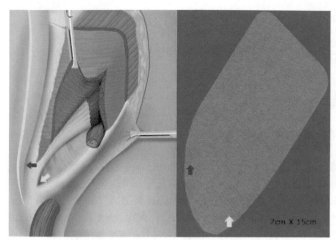

Fig. 1.2 Standard shape of the mesh. The narrow corner of the mesh fits into the angle between the inguinal ligament and the lateral border of the rectus sheath

based upon the definition used to identify this complication. However, rates of chronic pain that affects daily activity are in the 5% range and this complication should be discussed as part of the informed consent.

Mortality and morbidity related to inguinal hernia repair is unlikely, but with advanced age or severe comorbidities deaths may occur. Elective hernia surgery is a low-risk procedure with mortality rates of less than 0.1%. Emergency hernia operations carry a substantially higher mortality risk of approximately 1%. If bowel resection is performed, mortality rates may approach 10% [2–5].

In the clinic, patients are given a chlorhexidine wash to use the night prior or the morning of surgery. They are instructed not to shave the incision site as the microtrauma increases the risk of infection. Elderly patients or those with medical comorbidities undergoing elective repair undergo risk stratification and optimization prior to their operation.

1.1.2 Equipment

A sheet of prosthetic mesh measuring 7.5 × 15 cm is used. Monofilament, macroporous polypropylene meshes are preferred because their structure is more resistant to infection. Lightweight meshes have reduced rates of discomfort and pain with adequate tensile strength and equivalent recurrence rates [6]. The mesh should cover the entire floor of the inguinal canal. Its medial corner is tailored to its standard shape with a lower sharper angle to fit into the angle between the inguinal ligament and the rectus sheath and an upper wider angle to spread over the floor to the conjoined tendon where the rectus sheath and internal oblique aponeurosis meet (Fig. 1.2). In the case of a femoral hernia, the mesh may be modified to include a lateral triangular extension that is affixed to Cooper's ligament to exclude the femoral canal.

1.1.3   Patient Positioning

The patient is placed in the supine position on the operating room table.

1.1.4   Technique of Anesthesia

The procedure may be performed under local anesthesia with sedation as needed, which is our preferred choice for all reducible adult inguinal hernias. It is safe, simple, effective, economical, and without side effects such as nausea, vomiting, and urinary retention. Our choice of local anesthetic is a 50:50 mixture of 1% lidocaine (Xylocaine) and 0.5% bupivacaine (Marcaine) with 1/200,000 epinephrine. An average of 45 mL of this mixture is usually sufficient for a unilateral hernia repair. This is progressively administered in the following manner.

1.1.4.1 Subdermal Infiltration
Five mL of the 50:50 mixture is infiltrated along the line of the incision with a 25 gauge needle into the subdermal tissue parallel to the surface of the skin. Infiltration is continued as the needle is advanced, reducing the likelihood of intravascular infusion. This step blocks subdermal nerve endings and reduces the discomfort of intradermal infiltration, typically the most uncomfortable stage of local anesthesia.

1.1.4.2 Intradermal Injection and Creation of Skin Wheal
The needle that is in the subdermal plane is then withdrawn until the tip is in the intradermal level. The dermis is then slowly infiltrated with approximately 3 mL of the mixture along the line of the incision (Fig. 1.3).

1.1.4.3 Deep Subcutaneous Injection
Ten mL of the mixture is injected deep into the subcutaneous tissue through vertical insertions of the needle 2 cm apart. The needle is kept moving while injecting (Fig. 1.4).

1.1.4.4 Subaponeurotic Injection
Once the subcutaneous tissues are divided, 10 mL of the mixture is injected underneath the aponeurosis of the external oblique muscle through a window at the lateral aspect of the incision (Fig. 1.5). This injection floods the still enclosed inguinal canal and bathes all three major inguinal nerves with the mixture while the remainder of the subcutaneous tissues overlying the aponeurosis and canal are divided. The mixture also hydrodissects the canal lifting the external oblique aponeurosis away from the ilioinguinal nerve reducing the likelihood of nerve injury upon incising the aponeurosis. Occasional injection of the tissue near the pubic tubercle and around the neck and inside the indirect hernia sac is required to achieve complete local anesthesia. Additionally, splashing 10 mL of the mixture

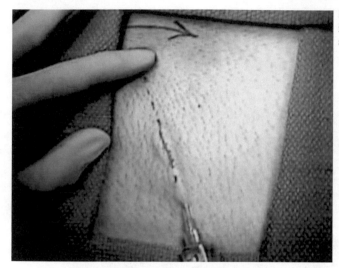

Fig. 1.3 Intradermal injection and creation of skin wheal

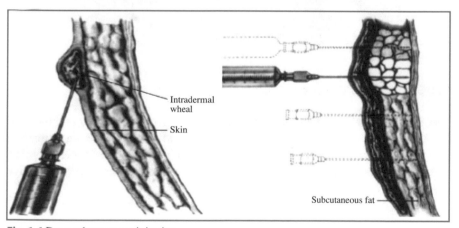

Fig. 1.4 Deep subcutaneous injection

into the canal before closure of the external oblique aponeurosis can further prolong the analgesic effect.

1.1.5 Sedation

Rapid, short-acting anxiolytic and amnestic agents such as propofol can be administered to mitigate the patient's anxiety and reduce to the amount of local anesthetic injected during the operation. If the hernia is not reducible, general or epidural anesthesia in addition to local infiltration of anesthetics is recommended.

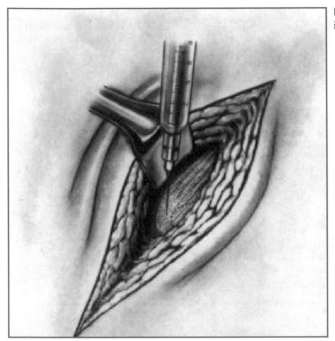

Fig. 1.5 Subaponeurotic injection

1.1.6   Operative Preparation

The patient is prepped with an antiseptic solution from above the umbilicus to the scrotum. The scrotum is prepped into the field if a large hernia extending into the scrotum is present. A dose of preoperative prophylactic antibiotic can be considered depending on practice patterns but is not required for clean, elective cases.

1.1.7   Incision and Exposure

A 5- to 6-cm skin incision starting from the pubic tubercle and extending laterally within the Langer line provides excellent exposure of the pubic tubercle and the internal ring.

1.1.8   Procedure

1. After skin incision, the external oblique aponeurosis is opened and its lower leaf is freed from the spermatic cord. The upper leaf of the external oblique is then freed from the underlying internal oblique muscle until the internal oblique aponeurosis is exposed. Separation of these layers exposes the

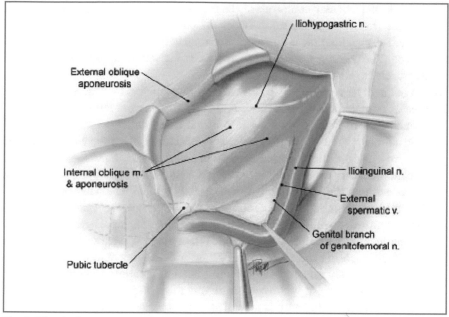

Fig. 1.6 Inguinal anatomy and identification of all three nerves

ilioinguinal and iliohypogastric nerves and creates ample exposure of the floor of the inguinal canal to accommodate the mesh prosthesis (Fig. 1.6). The mesh should overlap the internal oblique aponeurosis by at least 3 cm above the upper margin of the inguinal floor.

2. The cord with its cremasteric muscle covering is separated from the floor of the inguinal canal and the pubic bone for a distance of approximately 2 cm caudal to the pubic tubercle. When lifting the cord, care should be taken to include and preserve the ilioinguinal nerve and the visible blue external spermatic vein along with the cremasteric sheath. The genital nerve, which is always in juxtaposition to the external spermatic vessels, should be identified and preserved.

3. The cremasteric sheath is incised longitudinally at the level of the deep ring to explore the internal ring for an indirect hernia sac. Complete stripping and resection of the cremasteric fibers, described in the original version of the Lichtenstein repair, is unnecessary. The resultant direct exposure of the genital nerve, paravasal nerve fibers, and vas deferens to the mesh increases the risk of chronic groin pain and orchialgia.

4. An indirect hernia sac, if identified, is freed from the cord to a point beyond the neck of the sac may be inverted into the preperitoneal space without ligation. Ligation of the sac may cause of early postoperative nociceptive pain and does not affect the rate of recurrence. With a large hernia sac resection of the sac may be preferred to prevent pseudo-recurrence and to interrogate the preperitoneal space for a coexisting femoral hernia. Additionally, to minimize

the risk of testicular compromise, large, chronic, non-sliding scrotal hernia sacs are transected at the midpoint of the canal, leaving the distal section in place. The proximal sac is dissected proximal to the internal ring and is sutured ligated. The anterior wall of the distal sac is incised to prevent postoperative hydrocele formation.

5. Large direct hernia sacs may be inverted without tension to increase the surface area of contact between the mesh and floor of the canal and help prevent a pseudo-recurrence below the mesh. A broad based direct defect is imbricated with an absorbable running suture to approximate the transversalis fascia. A narrow necked direct hernia may be imbricated with a purse-string suture circumferentially along the transversalis fascia. These suture are specifically placed without tension carefully avoiding the inguinal ligament.

6. The femoral canal should be routinely evaluated via the space of Bogros through a small opening in the canal floor for a direct inguinal hernia or through the indirect sac with an indirect hernia. When present, the transversalis fascia is opened exposing the femoral canal and a coexisting femoral hernia may be simultaneously repaired using a modification creating a lateral triangular extension of the mesh with fixation of this mesh flap to Cooper's ligament. The flat portion of the mesh is then affixed in standard fashion.

7. A sheet of 7.5 × 15 cm of mesh shaped to cover the floor of the inguinal canal is sutured with a non-absorbable, monofilament suture material from the insertion of the rectus sheath to the pubic bone overlapping the symphysis by 1 to 2 cm caudally (Fig. 1.7). This is a crucial step in the repair because failure to cover this region with appropriate mesh overlap can result in recurrence of the hernia as the mesh contracts. The periosteum of the bone is avoided.

8. This suture is continued laterally with up to four passes to attach the lower edge of the patch to the inguinal ligament up to a point just lateral to the internal ring. Going further lateral risks injury to the femoral nerve. (Fig. 1.7) The depth of these bites should be carefully controlled to prevent injury or entrapment of the neurovascular structures passing deep to the inguinal ligament.

9. A slit is made at the lateral end of the mesh, creating two tails: a wide one (approximately 2/3 of the width) above and a narrower one (approximately 1/3 of the width) below. The wider upper tail is grasped with forceps and passed toward the head of the patient from underneath the spermatic cord; this positions the cord between the two tails of the mesh. The upper tail is crossed and placed over the narrower one and held with a hemostat (Fig. 1.8).

10. With the cord retracted downward and the upper leaf of the external oblique aponeurosis retracted upward, the upper edge of the patch is sutured in place with two or three interrupted absorbable sutures, one to the rectus sheath and the others to the internal oblique aponeurosis just lateral to the internal ring (Fig. 1.9). Suturing the upper edge of the mesh to the internal oblique muscle should be avoided to prevent injuring the intramuscular segment of the iliohypogastric nerve.

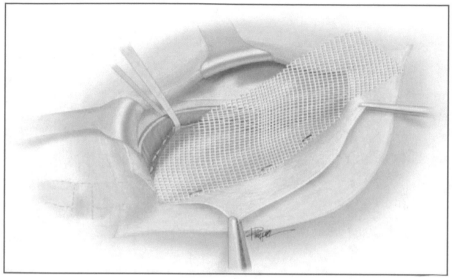

Fig. 1.7 Lateral fixation of mesh to the inguinal ligament with non-absorbable running suture. There is 1-2 cm overlap on the rectus muscle

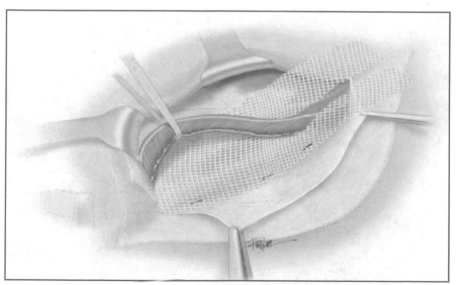

Fig. 1.8 A slit is made in the mesh laterally. The upper tail is 2/3 the width of the mesh and the lower tail is 1/3 the width of the mesh

11. Using a single non-absorbable monofilament suture, the lower lateral edges of each of the two tails are fixed to the inguinal ligament just lateral to the completion knot of the lower running suture, leaving adequate space for the passage of the spermatic cord and recreating the mesh internal ring (Fig. 1.10).

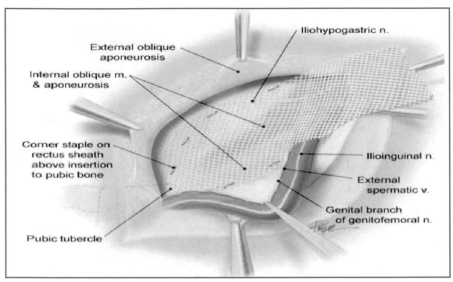

Fig. 1.9 Fixation of the upper border of the mesh to the internal oblique aponeurosis with interrupted, absorbable suture

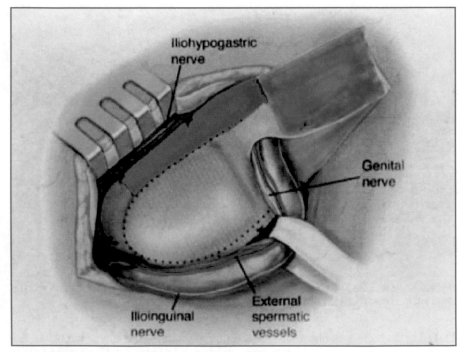

Fig. 1.10 The mesh is secured to the inguinal floor. Tails are sutured together with non-absorbable suture to recreate the internal ring. The tails should sit at least 5 cm lateral to the new internal ring underneath the external oblique aponeurosis

12. The excess patch on the lateral side is trimmed, leaving at least 5 cm of mesh beyond the internal ring to address any coexisting interstitial or low-lying Spigelian hernia. This is tucked underneath the external oblique aponeurosis, which is then closed over the cord with an absorbable suture.

1.1.9 Closure

Scarpa's fascia is reapproximated in interrupted fashion with an absorbable suture. The skin is closed with an absorbable subcuticular suture or staples.

1.1.10 Postoperative Care

Patients are instructed to avoid strenuous activity that significantly increases intra-abdominal pressure in the postoperative period for comfort but otherwise activity is unrestricted. Cardiovascular activity immediately following surgery is encouraged. Analgesic medications should be given to the patient. Patients are typically discharged home the same day.

1.2 Potential Complications

Recurrence rates for Lichtenstein hernia repair are uniformly low with most studies citing rates below 1% [2–5]. Rates of chronic pain vary with studies ranging from 0.5% to over 60% depending on the definition and means of measuring this outcome. Infection, bleeding, and ischemic orchitis are all low frequency events [7, 8]. Seroma and hematoma are typically expectantly managed with minimal morbidity. Visceral injury is rare but possible, especially in the incarcerated and strangulated scenario and with sliding or Richter's hernias. Urgent evaluation and operative management of these cases help to minimize systemic toxicity and risk.

1.3 Key Principles for Minimizing Recurrence and Postoperative Pain

In the mid 1990s, the Lichtenstein group made several modifications to the Lichtenstein technique, commonly referred to as the Amid-modified Lichtenstein repair, in order to align it with key principles that they identified as crucial to the success of the operation and comprising the technique described in this chapter [7].

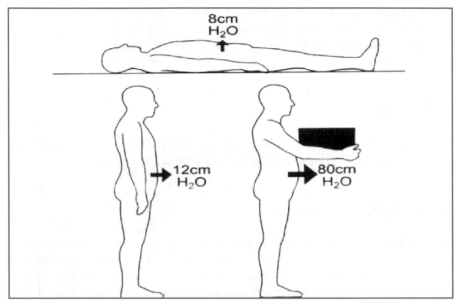

Fig. 1.11 Intra-abdominal pressure in various conditions

1.3.1 Intra-abdominal Pressure Gradient

Mean intra-abdominal pressure when a patient is supine is approximately 8 cm H_2O. This changes to 12 cm H_2O when standing and as high as 80 cm H_2O with straining and vomiting (Fig. 1.11). Elevated intra-abdominal pressure causes a protrusion of the lower abdominal wall, and in particular the transversalis fascia, anteriorly. Prosthetic based repairs must take this forward movement into consideration in order to be truly tension-free. An initial flaw was a mesh that was kept flat and therefore subject to tension with forward protrusion of the lower abdominal wall with elevated intra-abdominal pressures. The mesh was modified to have a slightly relaxed, tented, or domed shape in order to compensate for this protrusion and take tension off the mesh-tissue suture line.

1.3.2 Mesh Shrinkage

Reduction in mesh size after implantation is an important consideration in tension-free hernia repair. Studies from Lichtenstein's group and subsequently Klinge et al. demonstrated a 20% reduction in size in both transverse and craniocaudal directions after implantation [6, 7]. Construction of the mesh must therefore account for both reduction of its size and increased intra-abdominal pressures in order to remain tension-free once secured. The implications for an incorrectly sized and shaped mesh include recurrence, nerve entrapment, mesh migration, meshoma, and chronic postoperative pain.

In the initial description, the mesh did not extend beyond the pubic tubercle to overlap the pubic bone. It was also too narrow to provide adequate tissue contact with the inguinal floor in order to promote full tissue ingrowth and incorporation [8]. A standard size of 7.5×15 cm was recommended to provide both adequate laxity and surface area to accommodate intra-abdominal pressures and shrinkage (Fig. 1.1).

Identification and protection of the ilioinguinal, iliohypogastric, and genital branch of the genitofemoral nerve reduces the risk of nerve injury and entrapment with mesh placement. The practice of using continuous sutures to secure the top edge of the mesh was changed to interrupted sutures in order to minimize injury to the iliohypogastric nerve [8]. In some situations, this nerve abuts the upper border of the mesh and is at risk for entrapment. When this occurs, a slit can be made in the mesh to accommodate the aberrant course of the iliohypogastric nerve. In the same manner, the practice of "lesser cord" dissection of the genital nerve and lateral spermatic vessels off the cord with passage between a gap in the mesh-inguinal ligament suture line was also abolished [8].

1.3.3 Prosthesis Type

Adequate knowledge and appropriate use of prosthetic material is important to the success of a groin hernia operation. Mid to lightweight, macroporous, monofilament mesh is the prosthetic of choice. It allows for proper shape along with infiltration of fibroblasts, collagen fibers, blood vessels, and macrophages necessary for optimal incorporation of the mesh, strong and durable repair, and minimal complications. Mesh materials continue to evolve and ongoing refinement to address these key issues is essential to improve outcomes.

1.4 Modifications: Sutureless Fixation

Fixation in most inguinal hernia repair techniques remains a primary source of technical error potentially leading to inflammation, hematoma, injury, entrapment, and pain. Sutureless modifications to the Lichtenstein technique including fibrin or cyanoacrylate glue fixation and self-gripping meshes were developed in hopes of decreasing the incidence of chronic pain with similar recurrence rates. Level 1b evidence from a prospective randomized controlled study of fibrin glue, the Tissucol/Tisseel for Mesh fixation in Lichtenstein hernia repair (TIMELI) trial, compared fibrin glue to traditional suture fixation [9]. In this study, fibrin glue fixation was associated with significantly less postoperative pain at 1 and 6 months, providing a 45% reduction in chronic symptoms such as numbness, pain, and groin discomfort at one year. The 2015 FinnMesh multicenter randomized controlled trial compared cyanoacrylate glue, self-gripping mesh, and suture fixation found that cyanoacrylate glue had no appreciable benefit over suture fixation in terms of postoperative and chronic pain, and that self-gripping mesh demonstrated less pain only on the first postoperative day [10]. Though recurrence rates are equivalent to those of traditional suture fixation [9, 10], evidence is mixed for the benefits of atraumatic fixation methods as a whole. In patients with an increased risk of postoperative pain, these techniques may prove beneficial and should be considered.

1.5   Discussion

All surgeons that treat inguinal hernias should have detailed knowledge of groin anatomy and, based on the clinical situation, choose the technique that will best treat the patient contingent upon the expertise and preferred operative techniques of surgeon. In addition, they must understand the advantages and disadvantages of each technique as well as the appropriate indications.

The European Hernia Society (EHS) updated its consensus guidelines on the treatment of inguinal hernia in adults with best available data in 2014 [11]. As in 2009, the highest level of evidence (1A) and grade of recommendation (A) supports the use of the Lichtenstein tension-free hernioplasty for repair of primary, unilateral, symptomatic inguinal hernias. This technique is superior to the Bassini and Shouldice methods of tissue repair [2–5].

1.5.1   Lichtenstein versus Other Mesh-based Repairs

Prior comparison of the Lichtenstein technique to other mesh based repairs such as the Prolene Hernia System (PHS) and the Plug and Patch (PP) lacked adequate long-term data. The 2014 update included several RCTs and meta-analyses comparing PHS/Lichtenstein and PP/Lichtenstein with follow-up ranging from 1 to 4 years. Results for PP/Lichtenstein demonstrated a 5–10 minute decrease in operative time with no other appreciable benefits. PHS/Lichtenstein showed contradictory data on both operative time and perioperative complications. There were no differences with postoperative hematomas or infections. Both PHS and PP cost more than the mesh used for the Lichtenstein repair with no appreciable benefit [8]. In our practice and in the literature, we have seen migration of the plug causing chronic pain and in some instances, visceral, vascular, or bladder erosion. PHS placement involves entry into the preperitoneal space and may place the preperitoneal nerves and vas deferens at risk. Proper deployment is essential with meshoma and contraction seen from inadequate dissection and folding of the posterior leaflet.

1.5.2   Lichtenstein versus Laparoscopic Repair

The updated EHS guidelines maintain that for unilateral and bilateral primary inguinal hernias, the Lichtenstein repair is equivalent to the endoscopic approach with comparable recurrence rates [11]. However, the surgeon must be facile with the endoscopic approach to achieve equal results between the two techniques. The learning curve for endoscopic techniques is estimated to be 50–100 cases, with the first 30–50 being the most critical, whereas the Lichtenstein technique is easier to teach and replicate at all levels. Outcomes of non-experts and supervised residents performing the Lichtenstein repair for primary inguinal hernias are comparable to those of experts [11].

The open repair offers other distinct advantages over endoscopic repair. From a hospital system perspective, it is the most cost-effective procedure. However, from a socioeconomic standpoint, it is argued that endoscopic repair is more cost-effective for individuals who are actively participating in the labor market due to an earlier return to work [12]. In our experience, these differences are less pronounced with expectations and activity restrictions limiting patients more than physiologic impairment.

Open repair can be performed under local anesthesia and conscious sedation, obviating the stress and risk of general anesthesia and insufflation in patients who are at higher risk for complications. Both methods are demonstrably safe, though there is a higher potential risk of blood vessel and visceral organ injury with endoscopic techniques when compared to the Lichtenstein repair [13]. For a recurrent hernia after prior open operation, endoscopic repair is recommended over Lichtenstein repair since it accesses and unscarred plane resulting in less postoperative pain, faster recovery, and lower incidence of chronic pain [11].

1.5.3   Mesh Fixation

The 2014 EHS guidelines also address the method of mesh fixation in the Lichtenstein repair assessing atraumatic fixation with fibrin glue or cyanoacrylate glue. The TIMELI results favored fibrin glue fixation while cyanoacrylate glue had no appreciable benefit over suture fixation in terms of postoperative and chronic pain. Self-gripping mesh demonstrated less pain after the first postoperative day with no longer term benefits. Importantly, atraumatic fixation methods had recurrence rates equal to suture fixation at one year but at a higher cost than traditional suture fixation [11]. The update provides a Level B recommendation that atraumatic fixation can be used in Lichtenstein repairs with no adverse changes in recurrence rates at one year.

In our practice, we routinely offer the Amid-modified Lichtenstein tension-free hernioplasty or totally extraperitoneal endoscopic repair (TEP) for patients with primary, unilateral inguinal hernias. We counsel patients that both techniques have similar excellent outcomes and demonstrate no superiority in terms of chronic pain or recurrence. For those who wish to avoid general anesthesia, have increased cardiopulmonary risk, or prior lower abdominal surgery, the modified Lichtenstein technique can be performed with minimal operative risk and excellent outcomes. It is effective for all types of inguinal hernias. However, challenges do arise with femoral hernias or recurrent inguinal hernias after an anterior repair. While a female hernia can be repaired effectively with a Lichtenstein repair, a laparoscopic approach may be preferred given the higher incidence of femoral hernias. These patients, along with younger male patients who desire a faster convalescence and those with bilateral inguinal hernias, may benefit more from a laparoscopic repair.

1.6   Conclusions

The original intent of Lichtenstein was to "repair hernias without disability". In the past 30 years, refinement and proliferation of his techniques have dramatically improved patient outcomes. The Lichtenstein tension-free hernioplasty has been compared to numerous tissue and prosthetic inguinal hernia repairs and is either comparable or superior to all methods in terms of recurrence, postoperative pain, productivity time lost, chronic pain, complications, costs, and recurrence rates. It continues to be a gold standard operation for the repair of inguinal hernias.

References

1. Amid PK (2004) Lichtenstein tension-free hernioplasty: its inception, evolution, and principles. Hernia 8:1–7
2. McGillicuddy JE (1998) Prospective randomized comparison of the Shouldice and Lichtenstein hernia repair procedures. Arch Surg 133:974–978
3. Danielsson P, Isacson S, Hansen MV (1999) Randomized study of Lichtenstein compared with Shouldice inguinal hernia repair by surgeons in training. Eur J Surg 165:49–53
4. Nordin P, Bartelmess P, Jansson C et al (2002) Randomized trial of Lichtenstein versus Shouldice hernia repair general surgical practice. Br J Surg 89:45–49
5. Simons MP, Aufenacker T, Bay-Nielsen M et al (2009) European Hernia Society guidelines on the treatment of inguinal hernia in adult patients. Hernia 13:343–403
6. Amid PK (1997) Classification of biomaterials and their related complications in abdominal wall hernia surgery. Hernia 1:12–19
7. Klinge U, Klosterehalfen B, Muller M et al (1998) Shrinking of polypropylene mesh in vivo: an experimental study in dogs. Eur J Surg 164:965–969
8. Amid PK, Shulman AG, Lichtenstein IL (1993) Critical scrutiny of the open tension-free hernioplasty. Am J Surg 165:369–371
9. Campanelli G, Pascual MH, Hoeferlin A et al (2012) Randomized, controlled, blinded trial of Tisseel/Tissucol for mesh fixation in patients undergoing Lichtenstein technique for primary inguinal hernia repair: results of the TIMELI trial. Ann Surg 255:650–657

10. Rönkä K, Vironen J, Kössi J et al (2015) Randomized multicenter trial comparing glue fixation, self-gripping mesh, and suture fixation of mesh in Lichtenstein hernia repair (FinnMesh Study). Ann Surg 262:714–719 (discussion 719–720)
11. Miserez M, Peeters E, Aufenacker T et al (2014) Update with level 1 studies of the European Hernia Society guidelines on the treatment of inguinal hernia in adult patients. Hernia 18:151–163
12. Amid PK (2004) Causes, prevention, and surgical treatment of post-herniorrhaphy neuropathic inguinodynia: triple neurectomy with proximal end implantation. Hernia 8:343–349
13. Amid PK (2005) Groin hernia repair: open techniques. World J Surg 29:1046–1051

Tension-free, Sutureless Primary Inguinal Hernia Repair: the Trabucco Technique

2

Giampiero Campanelli, Piero Giovanni Bruni, Andrea Morlacchi, and Marta Cavalli

2.1 Introduction and Technical Background

The anatomically closed space in the inguinal canal below the external oblique aponeurosis (subaponeurotic space) was referred to as the "inguinal box" by Ermanno E. Trabucco (August 15, 1926 - March 9, 2015) in 1988 (Fig. 2.1) [1, 2, 3]. It had been noticed that the size and shape of this space has minimal variations from one individual to another: it measures around 12 cm from the anterosuperior iliac spine to the pubic tubercle, 7 cm from the anterosuperior iliac spine to the deep inguinal ring, 5 cm from the internal inguinal ring to the pubic tubercle, and 5 cm from the insertion of the external oblique muscle on the anterior sheath of the rectus muscle to the shelving edges of Poupart's ligament (Fig. 2.2).

The Trabucco technique is based on the utilization of a preshaped mesh in all primary inguinal hernia repairs. In other words, a universal preshaped mesh that will virtually always fit into the subaponeurotic inguinal space of every individual (Fig. 2.3) [1, 2, 4]. In order for a sutureless preshaped mesh to be effective, it must be sufficiently rigid and possess a controlled memory (to remain flat without a tendency to wrinkle or curl) [5].

This preshaped mesh consists of monofilament polypropylene weaved into a mesh structure. The mesh is then treated with a combination of heat and traction in order to tighten the weave and flatten the mesh. This process allows the mesh to lose part of its memory achieving a controlled memory [6] and acquire a flat shape, thus losing its tendency to curl or wrinkle. The dimensions of this preshaped mesh are based on the average size and shape of the subaponeurotic inguinal space,

G. Campanelli (✉)
General and Day Surgery Unit, Center of Research and High Specialization for the Pathologies of Abdominal Wall and Surgical Treatment and Repair of Abdominal Hernia, Istituto Clinico Sant'Ambrogio
Milan, Italy
e-mail: giampiero.campanelli@grupposandonato.it

G. Campanelli (Ed), *Inguinal Hernia Surgery*,
Updates in Surgery
DOI: 10.1007/978-88-470-3947-6_2, © Springer-Verlag Italia 2017

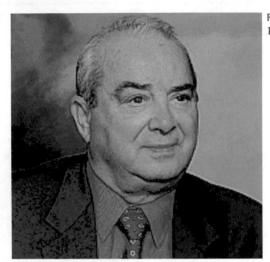

Fig. 2.1 Ermanno E. Trabucco (August 15, 1926 - March 9, 2015)

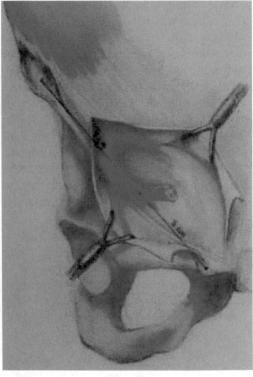

Fig. 2.2 The "inguinal box" (original drawing supplied by E.E. Trabucco) [1, 2]

which is 10 ± 4–5 cm. The mesh has a 1.2 cm wide circular opening for the exit of the spermatic cord. This opening is located 6 cm from the tip and 4 cm from the base of the mesh.

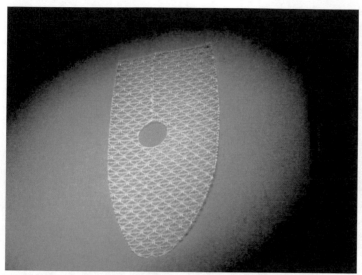

Fig. 2.3 Trabucco universal preshaped mesh

Meshes that are too soft placed on the floor of the inguinal canal without sutures will have a tendency to wrinkle or curl, thus increasing the potential for the formation of dead spaces and recurrences [6, 7]. Soft meshes cannot be implanted without sutures. All polypropylene prostheses have memory, even after sutures are applied.

In a sutureless technique, the mesh must lie flat when implanted and remain flat during the fibroblastic infiltration into its pores, a process that seals the mesh into place.

A sufficiently rigid preshaped mesh with controlled memory does not need to be sutured when placed into a closed space. Based on Pascal's principle, the intra-abdominal pressure is evenly distributed over a large surface area of mesh: the prosthesis will remain stretched uniformly in the inguinal box, without the need to be secured with sutures, it will always lie flat and will not move or form dead space.

Such a mesh is time saving and easy to implant. The postoperative discomfort is minimal and nerve injury rare. The identification and respect of the three nerves of the inguinal region is of crucial importance to reduce the rate of neuralgia in the short and long term [8].

The use of local anaesthesia requires that the surgeon properly recognize those nerves and respect them during the repair (Figs. 2.4 and 2.5). The intentional section of one or more nerves, when it is not possible to achieve a satisfactory nerve sparing, or special tricks to create tailored fenestrations (small windows) in the prosthesis to prevent scar tissue involving the spared nerves, ensure a further reduction of the rate of neuralgia and excellent patient outcomes [8].

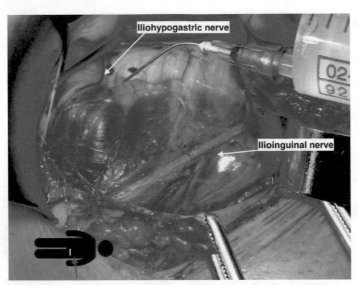

Fig. 2.4 Local anaesthesia during a Trabucco primary hernia repair: subfascial infiltration of iliohypogastric and ilioinguinal nerves

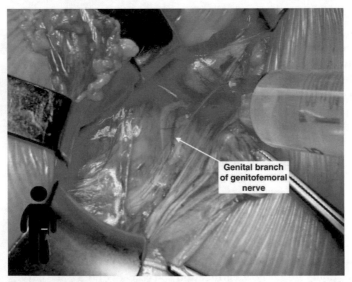

Fig. 2.5 Local anaesthesia during a Trabucco primary hernia repair: infiltration of genital branch of the genitofemoral nerve on the flattened floor of the inguinal box

The ideal polypropylene prosthesis for a tension-free primary inguinal hernia repair according to Trabucco must be as much as possible adapted to the patient himself; in particular, we have to consider the patient's constitution, age, gender, overall physical performance, personal daily needs and, of course, the type of hernia defect, which must be properly identified and typed before and during surgery.

All these parameters are reflected on the most appropriate choice of mesh to be used, and this can be done on the basis of its weight, thickness, porosity, rigidity, absence of memory and tendency to remain flat after implantation. The Hertra Herniamesh preshaped prosthesis (n. 1-6, from the most rigid to the softest meshes, which are ideal for athletes and young patients) developed by Trabucco [4] were never found to curl or to shrink after implantation [5] and, in our experience, are the best choice [3, 8].

Trabucco technique can be easily performed as a day case, under local anaesthesia, obtaining maximization of comfort for the patients, and is used routinely in all simple primary inguinal hernias [3].

The primary goal in the management of the patient with groin hernia is to repair the hernia while minimizing the incidence of postoperative complications, including recurrence. As with any surgical procedure, preoperative patient optimization is vital to reducing the risk of postoperative complications. This includes smoking cessation, control of diabetes mellitus, weight loss, maximization of nutritional status, establishing an exercise routine, and optimization of pulmonary and cardiac status.

2.2   Surgical Technique

After local anaesthesia [3, 8] (Fig. 2.6), a transverse incision is made 1 cm below the deep inguinal ring. The roof of the inguinal box is exposed and the external oblique aponeurosis (Fig. 2.7) is incised longitudinally. The cremaster muscle is grasped with two Allis forceps and opened longitudinally, while preserving the ilioinguinal nerve. The spermatic cord is lifted, exposing its mesentery. A Penrose drain encircles the mesentery and spermatic cord.

The femoral canal is explored for possible herniation by dissecting the lower crus from the cribriform fascia (Fig. 2.8). This dissection lengthens the crus, thus allowing a tension-free closure of the roof of the medial box.

Direct sacs are invaginated and flattened out with a tension-free prolene (or, better, polydioxanone, PDS) suture so that a preshaped mesh can be placed to lie flat on the floor of the medial box. Indirect sacs are carefully dissected and inverted through the internal ring (Fig. 2.9). Large deep inguinal rings are narrowed with sutures, if necessary.

After adequate dissection of the subfascial space, a small quantity of local anaesthetic or normal saline solution can be injected under the transversalis fascia near the deep inguinal ring so as to lift the fascia from the preperitoneum and create a fluid-filled space. The transversalis fascia is incised above the deep ring and around the spermatic cord and a subfascial space is developed with a finger.

A T4 flat plug (Fig. 2.10) can be positioned without sutures in the space under the fascia around the spermatic cord: its correct position must be visually verified. A T4 plug can also be inserted through a dilated internal inguinal ring

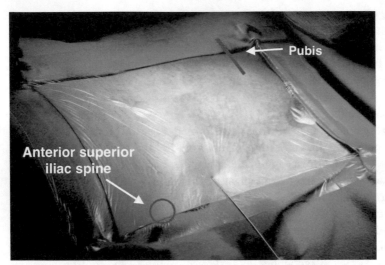

Fig. 2.6 Local anaesthesia before the inguinal incision, at the beginning of the procedure

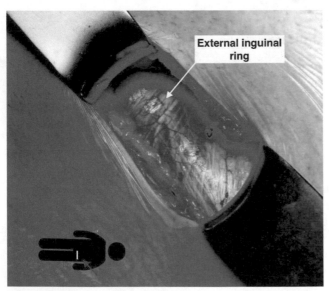

Fig. 2.7 Exposure of the external oblique aponeurosis

and positioned around the spermatic cord in the preperitoneal space (Fig. 2.11). At this step, it is suggested to invite the patient to strain to confirm that the plug has contained the hernia sac. The same plug can be used alone in small indirect inguinal hernias or, with a preshaped mesh in direct inguinal hernias to prevent indirect recurrences.

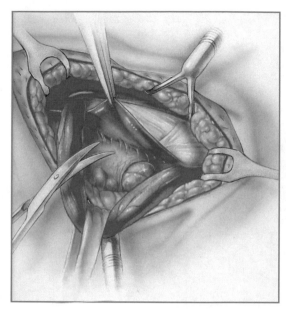

Fig. 2.8 Exploration of the femoral canal (original drawing supplied by E.E. Trabucco) [1, 2]

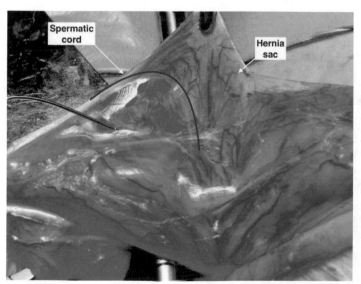

Spermatic cord

Hernia sac

Fig. 2.9 Isolation of indirect external oblique hernial sac

The medial end of the preshaped prosthesis is placed onto the dissected pubic tubercle and held in this position by an instrument. The mesh is placed on the flattened floor of the medial box with its hole surrounding the spermatic cord and its tails placed on the floor of the lateral box, under the aponeurosis of the external oblique muscle (Figs. 2.12 and 2.13).

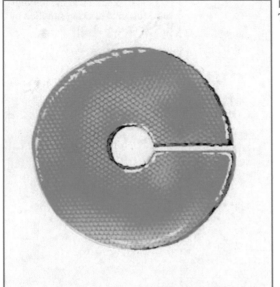

Fig. 2.10 T4 flat plug developed by Trabucco

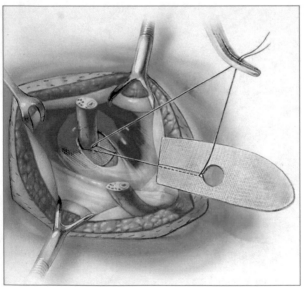

Fig. 2.11 T4 flat plug into a large internal inguinal ring, anchored to the preshaped onlay mesh (original drawings supplied by E.E. Trabucco) [1, 2]

The inguinal rings should not overlap, when the external oblique aponeurosis is closed behind the spermatic cord. Shifting a T4 plug lateral to the deep inguinal ring or the preshaped mesh toward the pubic tubercle prevents overlap of the inguinal rings and preserves the obliquity of the inguinal canal. For instance, in

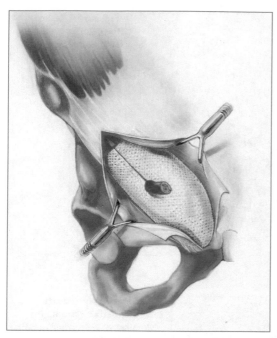

Fig. 2.12 Final view of a preshaped mesh in the inguinal box (original drawings supplied by E.E. Trabucco) [1, 2]

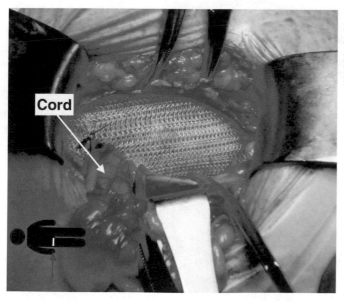

Fig. 2.13 Intra-operative final view of a polypropylene preshaped mesh implanted in the inguinal box

Cord

a medial box of 7 cm, the spermatic cord is pulled 1 cm medially, it exits from the hole of the preshaped prosthesis 1 cm medial to the deep inguinal ring, and overlaps the pubic tubercle by 1 cm [2].

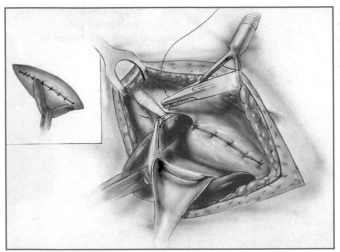

Fig. 2.14 Closure of the external oblique aponeurosis, under the spermatic cord (original drawing supplied by E.E. Trabucco) [1, 2]

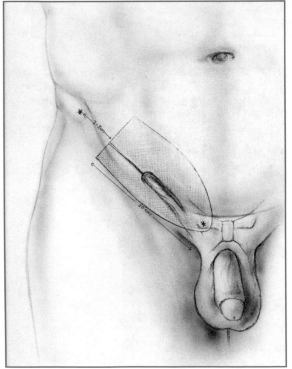

Fig. 2.15 Preshaped mesh superimposed on the anterior abdominal wall (original drawing supplied by E.E. Trabucco) [1, 2]

The external oblique aponeurosis is closed over the mesh, under the spermatic cord, and the procedure is complete (Figs. 2.14 and 2.15).

References

1. Trabucco EE (1993) The office hernioplasty and the Trabucco repair. Ann It Chir 44:127–149
2. Trabucco EE, Trabucco AF (1998) Flat plug and mesh hernioplasty in the "inguinal box": description of the surgical technique. Hernia 2:133–138
3. Campanelli G, Cioffi U, Cavagnoli R et al (1999) Open sutureless tension-free repair for primary inguinal hernia. Hernia 3:121–124
4. Trabucco EE, Trabucco AF, Rollino R et al (1998) Ernioplastica inguinale tension-free con rete presagomata senza suture secondoTrabucco. Minerva Chir 11:142–148
5. Petruzelli L (1999) Utilization of a rigid pre-shaped mesh according to the Trabucco technique: an experimental study. In: National Congress of SICADS. Ambulatory Surgery in Italy, Rome
6. Trabucco EE, Campanelli G, Cavagnoli R (1998) Nuove protesi erniarie in polipropilene. Minerva Chir 53:337–342
7. Amid PK (1987) Classification of biomaterials and their related complications in abdominal wall hernia surgery. Hernia 1:15–21
8. Alfieri S, Amid PK, Campanelli G et al (2011) International guidelines for prevention and management of post-operative chronic pain following inguinal hernia surgery. Hernia 15:239–249
9. Campanelli G, Cavagnoli R, Gabrielli F et al (1995) Trabucco's procedure and local anaesthesia in surgical treatment of inguinal and femoral hernia. Int Surg 80:29–34

Gilbert Technique of Inguinal Hernia Repair

3

Arthur I. Gilbert, Jerrold Young, and Rafael Azuaje

3.1 Introduction

The Gilbert technique of groin hernia repair has undergone generations of improvement since its inception in 1985 yet certain basic principles have been constant.

a. The myopectineal orifice (MPO), described by Fruchaud, is an area in the lower abdominal wall and groin that must be completely reinforced to repair currently presenting hernias and to prevent future hernias from forming in patients that create intraabdominal pressures during natural bodily functions and particularly in patients with chronic cough or prostatism.

b. The deep inguinal ring is actually a window in the muscular portion of the lower abdominal wall through which the spermatic cord emerges. Once the internal spermatic fascia covering the spermatic cord is opened the primary indirect peritoneal sac can be dissected free and invaginated into the preperitoneal space (space of Bogros).

c. The space of Bogros is a potential space that is easily actualized. It is the ideal space for placement of any barrier device (mesh or biologic) to protect the entire MPO. This pertains to repairs done by anterior or posterior open approaches as well as laparoscopic approaches using total extraperitoneal (TEP) or transabdominal preperitoneal (TAPP) techniques.

d. Tension on any repair produces unnecessary postoperative pain that can be long in duration and disabling. Tension in any repair, sutured or mesh, promotes the likelihood of recurrence.

e. Polypropylene mesh (PPM) is an excellent barrier material that is replicable in its manufacturing process and is tolerated well by tissues.

A.I. Gilbert (✉)
Miller-Miami Medical School, Hernia Institute of Florida
Miami, Florida, USA
e-mail: Bigart32@aol.com

G. Campanelli (Ed), *Inguinal Hernia Surgery,*
Updates in Surgery
DOI: 10.1007/978-88-470-3947-6_3, © Springer-Verlag Italia 2017

3.2   History

I was originally trained to do hernia repair using the modified Bassini repair. I used it through my surgical residency and for the following 14 years. In 1976 I changed to the Shouldice technique using polypropylene suture to do that three-layer repair. In 1984 I added a flat mesh patch to the Shoudice repair. It was placed in the preperitoneal space before the deepest tissues were sutured. In 1985 I added a rolled polypropylene plug repair sutured in the internal ring to repair all but very large indirect inguinal hernias. By 1986 I changed the rolled plug into a patch-like configuration that I passed through the deep inguinal ring into the space of Bogros. I added a patch of PPM to cover the medial triangle of the inguinal area. This repair became known as Gilbert's sutureless repair of inguinal hernias. Each of the components protects at separate levels and yet protects together. My final iteration, in 1997, is a hybrid of groin hernia repairs that I did prior to 1984, and since. The prolene hernia system (PHS) incorporates two flat polypropylene mesh patches, each of sufficient size to individually repair hernias protruding through the MPO. The two PPM patches are attached by a PPM connector which itself sits in the direct hernia defect of the posterior wall or the deep internal ring of an indirect hernia. The underlay patch mimics the posterior mesh repairs described earlier by Nyhus, Read and Stoppa, and used in TAPP and TEP laparoscopic repairs. The onlay mesh mimics the patch described by Usher and popularized by Lichtenstein. It reinforces the posterior wall and the deep inguinal ring. The connector is a version of the original rolled PPM plug I used to repair indirect inguinal hernias.

3.3   Gilbert Technique of Hernia Repair

The skin of the lower abdomen is prepped and draped. A generous amount of anesthetic solution is injected into the skin and subcutaneous layers. A 5-cm transverse incision is marked extending lateral from the pubic tubercle. The skin is incised and the subcutaneous layer is opened. Fifteen milliliters of additional anesthetic solution is infiltrated just beneath the external oblique aponeurosis (EOA). The cribiform fascia at the junction of the thigh is cleared. Inspection for a femoral hernia is done. The external ring is fully exposed. The EOA is opened through the external ring. Its medial flap is grasped with a clamp and is separated from the internal oblique fascia to actualize a space (Fig. 3.1). This is done at this step to avoid creating the wrong plane later. The ilioinguinal nerve is left undisturbed. The cremasteric fascia is opened and the spermatic cord is elevated. The leaves of the cremasteric fascia are separated from the cord. Its medial flap is excised. Its lateral flap that contains the cremasteric vessels and the genital branch of the genitofemoral nerve is preserved. The mesentery of the cord is opened to later accommodate the onlay patch. The transparent internal spermatic fascia that

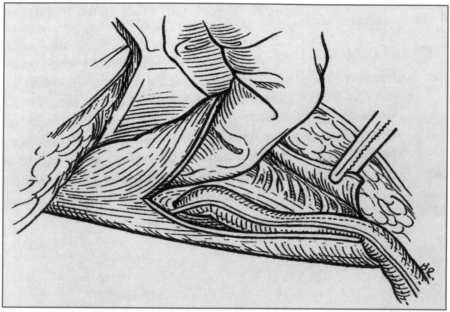

Fig. 3.1 Elevation of the external oblique aponeurosis develops the space for the onlay portion of the bilayer connected device (PHS). The anterior space is developed for the placement of the onlay patch of the PHS (reproduced with permission from J.E Fischer, D.B Jones, *Fischer's Mastery of Surgery*, 4th edn. © Lippincott Williams & Wilkins, 2011)

surrounds the spermatic cord is opened. If an indirect sac is identified and its distal part (head) is not firmly adherent to the cord, the sac is left intact and is dissected up to its true neck. If the sac's head is attached or scarred to the internal spermatic vessels, its mid-portion is divided leaving its distal portion in place. Its proximal portion is dissected up to its true neck and doubly ligated with a 2-0 Vicryl ligature. The proximal sac is invaginated through the deep inguinal ring. The posterior wall over the medial (Hesselbach's) triangle is inspected for a direct hernia or weakness.

For a lateral hernia the preperitoneal space is actualized by the surgeon passing a 4×4-opened sponge or an index finger through the deep inguinal ring and using it to push the fat and peritoneum away from the deep layer of the transversalis fascia (Fig. 3.2). The preperitoneal space is generously created to allow the underlay mesh to be fully deployed flat. After the head and neck of the sac have been fully dissected, it is invaginated through the deep ring (or, if preferred, the sac is ligated and divided). For direct hernias, the defective transversalis fascia is opened through the defect in the medial triangle and the preperitoneal space is actualized. The internal opening of the femoral canal and Cooper's ligament are visualized. The deep epigastric vessels are left intact except in cases of some pantaloon hernias that are better managed by dividing the vessels and converting the two

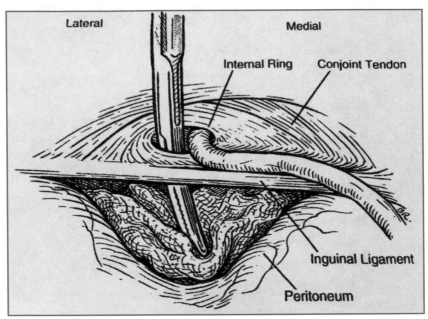

Fig. 3.2 For a lateral hernia the preperitoneal space of Bogros is actualized using an opened sponge (reproduced with permission from J.E Fischer, D.B Jones, *Fischer's Mastery of Surgery*, 4th edn. © Lippincott Williams & Wilkins, 2011)

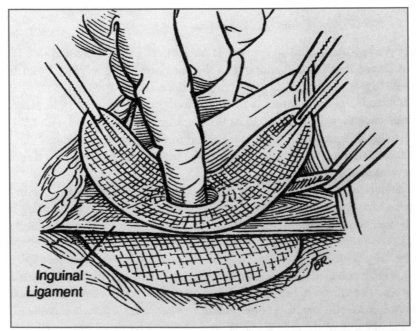

Fig. 3.3 The bilayer connected mesh device is placed in preparation to suture onlay patch (reproduced with permission from J.E Fischer, D.B Jones, *Fischer's Mastery of Surgery*, 4th edn. © Lippincott Williams & Wilkins, 2011)

defects into one. With the preperitoneal space sufficiently actualized by sponge and/or finger dissection the entire PHS device is inserted into the preperitoneal space (Fig. 3.3). Using a long forceps or one's forefinger, the edge of the circular underlay patch is deployed from its connector. The connector and onlay patch are extracted from the preperitoneal space. Holding the onlay like a bridle, lateral deployment of the circular underlay patch is facilitated. The technical goal of deployment is to spread the edge of the underlay patch circumferentially to be seated at maximum distraction from its connector. By doing so, the underlay patch fully covers the MPO superiorly, medially, and inferiorly ensuring coverage of the femoral canal. The underlay patch will become compressed against the abdominal wall, between the peritoneum and the transversalis fascia, by the patient's intraabdominal pressure. Typically, the internal ring is not tightened around the connector. The lateral flap of the onlay component is placed in the anterior space beneath the external oblique. Direct hernia defects are closed with one or two figure-of-eight sutures so that the connector will be comfortably seated and the underlay patch will be unable to get through the posterior wall.

The connector remains in the internal ring or in the direct defect. The medial part of the onlay patch is flattened against the transversus arch. The end of its medial leaf is loosely sutured 2 cm over the pubic tubercle. Effectiveness of the underlay patch alone can be evaluated by having the patent cough and perform a Valsalva maneuver before any sutures are placed in the onlay patch. In all cases of PHS repair the onlay patch should be sutured to the soft tissues (not into the periostium) over the pubic bone medial to the tubercle, at the middle of the transversus arch and at the middle of the inguinal ligament. To accommodate the spermatic cord through the onlay patch, a central slit is made close to the connector. The third suture is placed in the mid-portion of the inguinal ligament after the spermatic cord is accommodated. For the repair of an indirect hernia it is usually not necessary to suture the lateral flap that lies flat in the anterior space and is well covered by the EOA. For most direct hernias, a slit in the lateral flap of the onlay patch serves well to get mesh to protect the lateral triangle. The tails of the lateral flap are crossed and fixed with a single suture to prevent herniation through the slit. The patient again tests the repair by coughing and straining. Any excess of the onlay patch is excised. The spermatic cord and ilioinguinal nerve are replaced over the onlay patch. The EOA is closed with a 3-0 continuous Vicryl suture re-creating the external ring and being careful not to make it too tight. The subcutaneous layer is closed with 3-0 Vicryl sutures. Subcuticular closure with a 3-0 Vicryl Rapide suture is done. Dermabond is applied to the skin, making a swath approximately one-half to three-fourths of an inch on each side of the incision. The ends of the subcuticular suture are cut flush with the skin. A cover dressing is unnecessary.

The patient exercises in the operating room by doing bicycle motions. After sitting up on the operating table and moving from there to the gurney, the patient is retuned to the recovery room. After a light meal and being able to urinate, the patient leaves the ambulatory center about an hour after the operation. An ice bag, applied in the recovery area, is used for the remainder of the operative day. The patient is encouraged to ambulate often and to resume all activities (except driving for the first 48 hours) that are not uncomfortable. A Dulcolax suppository is given with the instruction to be used if the patient has not had a bowel movement by the next day.

Patients who live geographically close are encouraged to return in 4 to 7 days for a wound check. For those who live far away, we have a toll-free telephone number and encourage them to stay in contact regarding their progress. They are reminded they will have some ecchymotic discoloration (bruising) around the incision and scrotal skin and also some swelling. The bruising lasts approximately 10 days; the swelling lasts about 3 to 6 weeks. As the healing ridge becomes more prominent, it narrows and rises before it flattens.

Patients are recalled annually for re-evaluation of their repairs.

Suggested Readings

Gilbert AI (1989) An anatomic and functional classification for the diagnosis and treatment of inguinal hernia. Am J Surg 157:331–333
Gilbert AI (1997) Symposium on the management of inguinal hernias. Sutureless technique: second version. Can J Surg 40:209–212

Inguinal Hernia Repair Now and in the Future

4

John W. Murphy

4.1 Introduction

Inguinal hernia repair is one of the most common surgical procedures performed in the world today. Worldwide, hernia repairs account for some 2 million surgical cases per year, with 850,000 of those performed in the United States. An improved understanding of the underlying anatomical and physiological processes of hernia formation, and the widespread application of mesh products, have reduced the rate of hernia recurrence after primary repair to insignificant numbers.

To understand the foundation of this rapid and remarkable improvement in what used to be a quite complex and varied surgical technique, it is useful to consider three basic tenets in modern day hernia repair. These principles have been elucidated and refined over a 40-year period, occasionally meeting significant resistance from the "conventional wisdom" of the surgical community. Nevertheless, they have formed the basis of a common conceptual framework that has allowed the development of simple, rapid and permanent repair techniques for multiple forms of abdominal wall defects.

4.2 Past Advances

Read proposed that inguinal hernias formed as the result of a hitherto unknown disease process, rather than heavy lifting, coughing or a patent process vaginalis. He further proposed that abnormal collagen lay at fault, as well as noting a significant correlation between tobacco use and inguinal hernia incidence in a population of Veterans Administration patients. He attributed this to a protease-antiprotease imbalance seen in patients with pulmonary emphysema [1]. He postulated that this imbalance caused similar changes in the connective tissue of

J.W. Murphy (✉)
William Beaumont Hospital-Troy
Bloomfield Hills, Michigan, USA
e-mail: jmurphymd@earthlink.net

G. Campanelli (Ed), *Inguinal Hernia Surgery,*
Updates in Surgery
DOI: 10.1007/978-88-470-3947-6_4, © Springer-Verlag Italia 2017

the groin and termed this "metastatic emphysema". Weitz further solidified this theory when he demonstrated the presence of increased levels of active neutrophil elastase in smokers [2].

The main fibrillary components of dense connective tissue, including deep fascia, consist of collagen type I and collagen type III. Within the tissue matrix, heavy, inflexible collagen I fibers provide strength and resistance to deformation, while the lighter collagen III fibers, which provide elasticity, arise in a random arrangement. In the normal fascia, collagen I should exceed collagen III by a ratio of 3:1. Hernia patients exhibit an inverse ratio of collagen I to collagen III, as well as a decrease in collagen I generally; this abnormality results in a weakened and attenuated fascia, which can easily be compromised to form a hernia [3]. Pans published a series of biomechanical tests in which samples of transversalis fascia taken from patients with direct inguinal hernias demonstrated increased elasticity and maximal distention compared to controls, confirming the hypothesis that abnormal connective tissue was involved in the genesis of hernias [4]. The final advance in the histopathological theory of hernia formation lay in the understanding of the biochemical aspects of the collagen fibers themselves. An increase in matrix metalloproteinase, which degrades other types of collagen as well as other matrix components, has been observed in patients with direct inguinal hernias [5].

Anatomically, Fruchaud first described the myopectineal orifice (MPO), consisting of three potential zones of structural weakness in the inguinal region through which a hernia could form [6]. He also correctly observed that if these three areas were not covered in the initial repair, the chance of recurrence increased significantly.

Lastly, the use of implantable mesh as an abdominal wall prosthesis was first described half a century ago, but has only seen widespread acceptance in hernia repair in the last 25 years. Today, there are over 50 different mesh hernia devices on the market, each with several claimed benefits. The physico-mechanical properties of these meshes and their roles in the wound healing process have not been well understood until relatively recent years [7]. With a better understanding of these properties, it may be possible in the near future to "customize" the mesh for individual patients resulting in better outcomes [8].

For a decade or more, these concepts were debated at annual American and European Hernia Society meetings. It was only after Schumpelick declared that Read was "once a sinner and now a saint" that the concepts were fully accepted and a much better understanding of hernia formation was achieved.

4.3   Present Practice

The improvement in surgical outcomes since adoption of these three tenets has been undeniable. However, naysayers continue to proliferate today. Consider the continued popularity of tension (tissue) hernia repair. Based on our current physiological understanding of the tissue abnormality underlying hernia formation, it should logically follow that no amount of suturing abnormal tissue to abnormal tissue will create a repair of normal tissue strength. However, many surgeons continue performing these repairs and advocating for their application, either out of respect for what they learned in residency, or out of ignorance of the current literature.

The problem of quality surgical education also plagues hernia repair, just as it does every other area of general surgery. Many surgeons do not recognize, or were never taught, the significance of the MPO or the disease process behind hernia formation. This problem is exacerbated by a low research literacy rate and low attendance at research conferences within the surgical community. Low surgical volume also poses a problem; no matter what repair technique our hypothetical general surgeon applies or how studiously he or she reviews it, on average he or she will only perform about 50 of those repairs per year, not nearly enough to maintain competency.

Despite all these concerns, recurrence no longer significantly complicates modern day hernia repairs. The most significant complication in hernia repair today is chronic groin pain [9]. Various studies have placed the incidence of chronic groin pain following inguinal hernia repair at between 10 and 40%. With 850,000 hernia repairs performed in the U.S. annually, one can derive an absolute minimum of 85,000 affected patients per year – enough to fill any of the world's largest sporting venues to seated capacity. However, very few surgeons admit to having patients with chronic groin pain, or even seeing the complication at all. This apparent incongruity can be explained by a brief visit to any pain management clinic. The anesthesiologists who run these clinics will readily acknowledge that they see patients with chronic groin pain caused by hernia repair every single day. Generally the patient returns to the surgeon for a post-operative follow-up visit and complains of pain, which the surgeon dismisses as common acute post-operative pain and reassures the patient that the pain will improve by the next post-op visit. However, the next post-op visit comes and goes with the same pain complaint from the patient and the same reassurance from the surgeon, with no further action taken. The pattern continues until the patient, who is still in pain, becomes frustrated and returns to his/her primary care physician, who then issues a referral to the pain clinic. The surgeon in most cases remains unaware of this outcome, as neither the primary care physician nor the pain management anesthesiologist may want to risk offending a referral source by writing a formal letter to the surgeon.

In June 2011, the European Hernia Society published the International Guidelines for the Prevention and Management of Post-Operative Chronic Groin Pain [10]. This document represents a landmark achievement, in that it codified a definition of chronic groin pain, which is now stated as any groin pain lasting more than three months following inguinal hernia repair. Before the guidelines, "chronic groin pain" suffered from a myriad of occasionally conflicting descriptions, which posed significant difficulty in comparing data sets within the literature. Now, with an accepted definition in hand, efforts can be turned toward understanding causes, reducing incidence and improving outcomes.

Nerve damage, the use of mesh for the repair, and fixation of the mesh have all been postulated as causes of chronic groin pain. Nerve damage can result from direct trauma, stretching, vascular injury, and fixation. Mesh products, particularly if placed in the anterior space, may cause groin pain through incorporation of the mesh, resulting in either direct or indirect contact with nerves. Extensive dissection needed for placement of an anterior mesh may also play a role in post-op pain. Fixation of the mesh may cause groin pain by direct nerve entrapment, or by causing traction on smaller nerve branches as the mesh becomes incorporated. If fixation is required, absorbable sutures should be used.

Many of the causes mentioned above can be avoided by not placing mesh in the anterior space. By avoiding mesh in the anterior space, the dissection can be limited to identifying the defect, leaving the nerves in place, and performing the repair in the preperitoneal space.

Placing the mesh in the preperitoneal space still represents a fringe position, despite decades of evidence demonstrating the safety and efficacy of this approach. Most mesh products to date have been placed in the anterior space, but this is solely a matter of convenience rather than good biomechanics. Consider a flat tire, by way of analogy: it is of course easier to patch the outside of the tire, but the flat will recur as soon as the tire is inflated, as air pressure will force the patch away from the defect. Placing the patch inside the tire creates a permanent repair that will not succumb to air pressure, and indeed is reinforced by it. By this logic, the only reasonable places to implant mesh would be preperitoneal and intraperitoneal (as in laparoscopic repair), as both techniques take advantage of intra-abdominal pressure to reinforce the defect. However, many surgeons are not familiar with the preperitoneal space, and pose concerns ranging from incidence of bleeding to lack of sufficient volume to hold mesh. A quick review of anatomy allays both of these fears: there are no significant vessels anywhere within the preperitoneal space, and the space extends from the pubic tubercle to the diaphragm, and is routinely used to hold transplanted kidneys (which, of course, are orders of magnitude larger than any mesh prosthesis). The preperitoneal space also holds the advantage of not containing any nerves that can be entrapped or impinged upon by mesh, which in turn greatly reduces the incidence of chronic groin pain.

4.4   Future Advances

Our attention now turns to the use of robotic systems in inguinal hernia repair. In 2014, 570,000 robotic surgical procedures were done worldwide. This represents an increase of 179% since 2009. While gynecologic and urologic procedures seem to have plateaued, general surgical procedures under robotic assistance increased fourfold to 150,000 since 2009. One in four U.S. hospitals owns or leases a robot, representing 67% of installed robots and 79% of robotic procedure volume worldwide. Just as the number of robotic procedures has increased, so has the cost of the robot, from $900,000 for the original device to $2.3 million for the latest models. In addition, disposables costs run to $1 million per year per robot. In total, the use of the robot adds approximately $3,000-$6,000 incremental cost per procedure, regardless of procedure type. To date, there has been no significant clinical evidence that clinical outcomes or quality of care are improved.

A clear parallel can be drawn to the advent of laparoscopic repairs. When first proposed, laparoscopic inguinal hernia repair cost significantly more in equipment and disposables, required longer operating times, and had a very long learning curve. The same arguments have been put forward for robotic repairs and rightfully so. However, robotic repairs do offer some advantages over laparoscopic repairs. The picture is 3-D, does not move unless the operator wants, allows for easier dissection, and offers some improvement in surgeon ergonomics. Whether this repair offers any clear advantages over traditional laparoscopic repair, or over any of the minimally invasive open mesh repairs, remains to be explored.

In the more distant future, the entire question of surgical hernia repair may well become academic. A first step may be the development of simple assays which demonstrate the specific collagen metabolism of a patient.

Mesh implantation generally produces a predictable fibrotic response. But what mesh to use? Should it be large pore, small pore, absorbable, non-absorbable, coated, non-coated? Further studies can help elucidate the answers to these questions, and allow for tailoring the choice of mesh to the individual patient's biomarkers and tissue type. There also may be some potential for pharmaceutical stimulation of the wound healing process such as growth factors or protease inhibitors. Experimental studies have shown that the implantation of type I collagen-soaked sponges with seeded fibroblasts or fibroblast growth factor raises collagen deposition and increases the tensile strength of the wound [11].

In order to move forward, we must deal with what we know and can do now. We know that hernia formation in most cases is the result of a collagen deficiency, and not the result of wall strain. We know that apposing abnormal tissue to abnormal tissue results in a higher recurrence rate. We know that mesh repair techniques will reduce the incidence of recurrence, particularly if the mesh covers the entire myopectineal orifice. However, the use of mesh has resulted in an increased incidence of chronic groin pain, which is now the most common complication of inguinal hernia repair and must be addressed. An increasing weight of evidence demonstrates that placing the repair in the preperitoneal space reduces the incidence of chronic groin pain. These and other techniques may help us build the "bridge" of procedural knowledge that allows us to finally eliminate the problem of inguinal hernia.

References

1. Read RC (1995) Blood protease/antiprotease imbalance in patients with acquired herniation. Prob Gen Surg 12:41–46
2. Weitz JI, Crowley KA, Landman SL (1987) Increased neutrophil activity in cigarette smokers. Ann Int Med 107:680–682
3. Bellon JM, Bujan J, Honduvilla NG et al (1997) Study of biochemical substrate and role of metalloproteinase in fascia transversalis from hernia processes. Eur J Clin Invest 27:510–516
4. Pans A, Pierard GE, Albert A (1999) Immunohistochemical study of the rectus sheath and transversalis fascia in adult hernia. Hernia 3:45–51
5. Agren MS, Jorgensen IN, Andersen M et al (1998) Matrix metalloproteinase 9 level predicts optimal collagen deposition during early wound repair in humans. Br J Surg 85:68–71
6. Fruchaud H (1955) Anatomie chirurgicale des hernies de l'aine. Doin, Paris
7. Deeken CR, Abdo MS, Frisella MM, Matthews BD (2011) Physicomechanical evaluation of polypropylene, polyester, and polytetrafluoroethylene meshes for inguinal hernia repair. J Am Coll Surg 212:68–79
8. Deeken CR, Thompson DM, Castle RM, Lake SP (2014) Biaxial analysis of synthetic scaffolds for hernia repair demonstrates variability in mechanical anisotropy, non-linearity, and hysteresis. J Mech Behav Biomed Mater 38:6–16
9. Cunningham J, Temple WJ, Mitchel P et al (1996) Cooperative hernia study: pain in the postrepair patient. Ann Surg 224:598–602
10. Alfieri S, Amid PK, Campanelli G et al (2011) International guidelines for prevention and management of post-operative chronic pain following inguinal hernia surgery. Hernia 15:239–249
11. Marks MG, Doillon C, Silver FH (1991) Effects of fibroblasts and basic fibroblast growth factor on facilitation of dermal wound healing by type I collagen matrices. J Biomed Mater Res 25:683–696

3D Dynamic Anterior Repair: ProFlor Technique

5

Giampiero Campanelli, Andrea Morlacchi, Piero Giovanni Bruni, and Marta Cavalli

5.1   Introduction

If we look at the history of hernia repair, recurrences and complications are still a major problem for surgeons. During recent decades, many improvements have been attempted to reduce discomfort and chronic pain after surgery, but these still remain frequent [1]. The ProFlor hernia system was introduced with the aim of addressing such problems. It is designed for preperitoneal sutureless inguinal hernia repair. As already shown by some studies, a fixation-free preperitoneal repair leads to a significant reduction in chronic groin pain by reducing the risk of nerve damages or entrapment [2–4]. In addition to this, the particular structure of this device makes a physiological repair possible.

5.2   Device Characteristics

Despite the fact that the inguinal region is one of the most mobile parts of the human body, commonly used flat meshes for inguinal hernia are static devices which only strengthen the groin area by inducing the ingrowth of inelastic scar tissue. The idea behind the 3D Dynamic implant is that the inguinal region should be repaired preserving the physiological resistance to kinetic stresses of this region.

G. Campanelli (✉)
General and Day Surgery Unit, Center of Research and High Specialization for the Pathologies of Abdominal Wall and Surgical Treatment and Repair of Abdominal Hernia, Istituto Clinico Sant'Ambrogio
Milan, Italy
e-mail: giampiero.campanelli@grupposandonato.it

G. Campanelli (Ed), *Inguinal Hernia Surgery,*
Updates in Surgery
DOI: 10.1007/978-88-470-3947-6_5, © Springer-Verlag Italia 2017

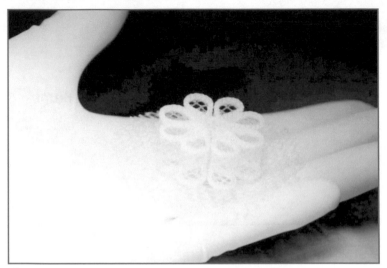

Fig. 5.1 The device with its central core and preperitoneal layer

The device is made of lightweight large-pore polypropylene and has a particular shape that, rather than just covering it, actually fills the defect. It has a preperitonal disk and a central multilamellar core that gives radial resilience, which explains why the implant stays inside the defect without needing any fixation [5] (Fig. 5.1).

Because of its geometrical structure, this device transforms expulsion forces into gripping forces, a key point of this sutureless repair. These forces lead to a better quality in tissue ingrowth, compared to other static meshes that are usually incorporated in a scar plate. This prolonged, low-load, cyclical stress to the abdominal wall seems to be the main cause of the obliteration of the defect and incorporation of the device with good quality tissue [6]. This entails less mesh shrinkage, as a result of the fact that the tissue covers the Freedom inguinal hernia device gradually, in a more physiological manner, unlike the case with commonly used polypropylene meshes that induce an acute fibrotic response. This may lead to a reduction in recurrence rate and patient discomfort [7].

5.3   Patient Selection

Almost every patient eligible for elective surgery for primary inguinal hernia could be selected for this kind of repair. Patients can be males or females, they should have a clinically relevant primary inguinal hernia with a defect size at operation between 20 and 35 mm in diameter, which corresponds to a M2/L2 in the European Hernia Society (EHS) groin hernia classification [8], and they should be diagnosed with direct or indirect defect.

Contraindications for this repair are: previous surgery on the hernia operative site, giant inguinoscrotal hernia, recurrent inguinal hernia, known collagen disorder, femoral hernia, body mass index >35, and cases in which peritoneum cannot be closed.

5.4 Surgical Technique

This procedure can be performed under local anesthesia and the patient can be discharged the same day of the operation.

After a horizontal skin incision of 3–6 cm, perform a dissection through the Scarpa's fascia to external oblique aponeurosis. Then expose the external inguinal ring and external oblique aponeurosis, open the aponeurosis and dissect and elevate the cord, in order to define whether the defect is direct or indirect. The procedure is slightly different for each kind of hernia.

For an *indirect defect*, identify the internal inguinal ring and remove all the adhesions and scar tissue around it. Dissect the sac from the cord structures up to the internal inguinal ring, isolating it circumferentially. Identify the nerves of the region, taking care not to damage or stretch them. After that, reduce the sac through the ring without ligating it because it may cause initial or chronic pain. Finally, dissect with a finger the parietal peritoneum from the posterior abdominal wall, creating enough room to accommodate the preperitoneal disc of the implant (Fig. 5.2).

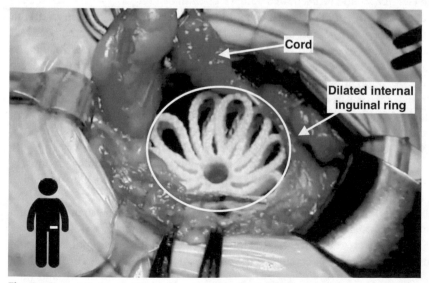

Fig. 5.2 Correct device positioning in a case of indirect defect

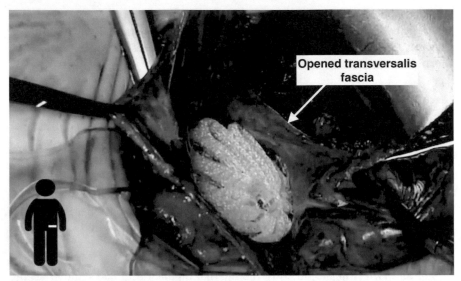

Opened transversalis fascia

Fig. 5.3 Correct device positioning in a case of direct defect

For a *direct defect*, dissect the sac from abdominal wall structures, paying attention to the nerves, removing adhesions and scar tissue around the hernia. Then open the transversalis fascia, with an incision as wide as necessary to detach the sac from the posterior wall. Dissect the parietal peritoneum with a finger and then check the integrity of the peritoneum (Fig. 5.3).

After having identified and isolated the defect, choose the size of the implant: a 25-mm device should be used for a defect of less than a finger, a 40-mm device for a defect of two fingers. The implant should be folded around the core and then put into the delivery device, aligning the space between the loops with the notch on the flange of the device. This is important for indirect hernias because it helps the loops fold open around the cord. Use the Freedom inguinal hernia delivery device to place the implant into the hernia defect (Fig. 5.4). Gently push the device into the defect, dilating it, until the flange rests on the external border of the defect. Release the implant by pushing the plunger, and then remove the delivery device. If needed, the freedom inguinal hernia implant can be adjusted using forceps, to allow adequate placement of the preperitoneal disk. Be careful not to apply excessive strength during this maneuver because it may lead to damage to muscle fibers or bleeding. After delivery, the implant should be placed into the defect with the loops forming a complete circle and the disk lying in the preperitoneal space, parallel to the posterior wall of the inguinal canal. In the case of an indirect defect, the spermatic cord should be between two of the loops.

Prior to closure, appropriate positioning and stability of the implants should be confirmed by a patient cough test if under local anesthesia or by gently pulling

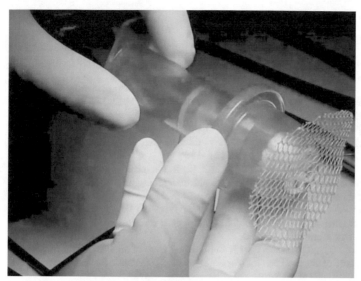

Fig. 5.4 Implant folded inside the delivery device

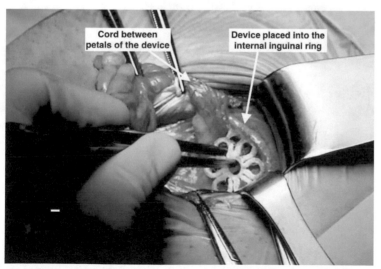

Fig. 5.5 The stability of the device should always be checked by gently pulling it with a forceps

out the implant to verify if proper resistance is present (Fig. 5.5). Then close the external oblique, leaving the cord in its natural subfascial position, and Scarpa's fascia. Close the wound using standard surgical technique. Usually, no drain is needed.

References

1. Kim-Fuchs C, Angst E, Vorburger S et al (2012) Prospective randomized trial comparing sutured with sutureless mesh fixation for Lichtenstein hernia repair: long-term results. Hernia 16:21–27
2. Campanelli G, Cavalli M, Biondi A, Bombini G (2014) Approccio posteriore open - TOP Total Open Preperitoneal (modified Wantz repair). In: Greco VM (ed) Guida alla chirurgia tailored dell'ernia inguinale. EdiSES, Napoli, pp 135–141
3. Sajid MS, Craciunas L, Singh KK et al (2013) Open transinguinal preperitoneal mesh repair of inguinal hernia: a targeted systematic review and meta-analysis of published randomized controlled trials. Gastroenterol Rep (Oxf) 1:127–137
4. Campanelli G, Pascual MH, Hoeferlin A et al (2012) Randomized, controlled, blinded trial of Tisseel/Tissucol for mesh fixation in patients undergoing Lichtenstein technique for primary inguinal hernia repair: results of the TIMELI trial. Ann Surg 255:650–657
5. Amato G, Agrusa A, Romano G et al (2014) Modified fixation free plug technique using a new 3D multilamellar implant for inguinal hernia repair: a retrospective study of a single operator case series. Hernia 18:243–250
6. Amato G, Romano G, Agrusa A et al (2015) Biologic response of inguinal hernia prosthetics: a comparative study of conventional static meshes versus 3D dynamic implants. Artif Organs 39:E10–23
7. Amato G, Lo Monte AI, Cassata G et al (2011) A new prosthetic implant for inguinal hernia repair: its features in a porcine experimental model. Artif Organs 35:E181–190
8. Miserez M, Alexandre JH, Campanelli G et al (2007) The European hernia society groin hernia classification: simple and easy to remember. Hernia 11:113–116

Total Open Preperitoneal (TOP) Technique (modified Wantz)

6

Giampiero Campanelli, Piero Giovanni Bruni, Andrea Morlacchi, and Marta Cavalli

6.1   Introduction

Stoppa proposed the open posterior preperitoneal repair for the first time in 1965 [1, 2], under the name of "giant prosthetic reinforcement of the visceral sac" (GPRVS). Later, in 1989 Wantz [3] proposed a similar procedure, differing from the Stoppa technique for a unilateral repair.

In both procedures, a large bilateral Dacron mesh was placed in the preperitoneal space, covering Fruchaud's myopectineal orifice with extensive overlap in all directions so that the peritoneal sheet could not be extended.

The myopectineal orifice is the weak spot where all hernias of the groin begin; it is covered only by the transversalis fascia and includes the Hesselbach's triangle, the deep inguinal ring and the Scarpa's triangle of the femoral region [4]. A mesh placed in this space is compressed by the internal abdominal pressure and fixed against the internal abdominal wall, in accordance with Pascal's hydrostatic principle: when there is an increase in pressure at any point in a confined fluid, there is an equal increase at every other point in the container.

The posterior preperitoneal approach provides an alternative to the anterior preperitoneal approach which, in cases of recurrent herniation, encounters scarring, possibly leading to damage to the spermatic cord, nerves, and blood vessels. Moreover, this approach permits a complete and clear view of both inguinal and femoral regions.

Few data are present in the literature with regard to the Stoppa and Wantz techniques, which demonstrates that they did not have success among general

G. Campanelli (✉)
General and Day Surgery Unit, Center of Research and High Specialization for the Pathologies of Abdominal Wall and Surgical Treatment and Repair of Abdominal Hernia, Istituto Clinico Sant'Ambrogio
Milan, Italy
e-mail: giampiero.campanelli@grupposandonato.it

G. Campanelli (Ed), *Inguinal Hernia Surgery*,
Updates in Surgery
DOI: 10.1007/978-88-470-3947-6_6, © Springer-Verlag Italia 2017

Table 6.1 Recurrent hernia classification by Campanelli

Type	Localization	Features	Technique
R1	Near the internal inguinal ring	First recurrence, reducible, thin patient, wall defect <2 cm	Gilbert with plug repair
R2	Above the pubic tubercle	First recurrence, reducible, thin patient, wall defect <2 cm	TOP
R3	Whole inguinal wall defect	Multirecurrence and/or irreducible and/or extended wall defect, femoral recurrence	TOP

surgeons, probably because they are more difficult than the anterior preperitoneal approach and require excellent knowledge of the anatomy and extensive experience in the surgery of this region [5]. Another reason could be that they lost appeal with the advent of the laparoscopic approach in the early 90s.

After a long-standing experience in abdominal hernia repair, we propose a modified open posterior preperitoneal approach, called TOP (Total Open Preperitoneal) technique, that we usually use for the repair of giant inguinal hernia [6], recurrent inguinal hernia [7, 8], femoral hernia or in the treatment of postoperative chronic pain [9].

According to our original classification for recurrent inguinal hernia (Table 6.1), based on the location of the recurrent defect and on the patient's features, we suggest the TOP technique for the following hernias:

- R2: first recurrence, after plastic or prosthetic repair, medial (direct) reducible hernia with a small (<2 cm) defect above the pubic tubercle in a thin patient (possible also under local anaesthesia);
- R3: large defect (inguinal eventration) or multi-recurrent hernias or non-reducible recurrent hernia.

6.2   Technique

The TOP technique can be done under local, spinal or general anaesthesia (the last of these is suggested during the learning curve) and requires a 5-8-cm-long suprapubic transverse lateral incision, 2 cm below the superior-anterior iliac spin (ASIS) (Fig. 6.1) [3, 10].

After the subcutaneous space is cut, the external oblique muscle and rectus muscle aponeurosis are opened together and the fibers of the internal oblique and transversus muscle are split laterally (Fig. 6.2) [3, 10]. At this level it is sometimes possible to detect the ilioinguinal and iliohypogastric nerves: during the procedure for the treatment of chronic postoperative pain, these are tied, cut and buried in muscle (Fig. 6.2) [9].

A retractor is placed so that the rectus muscle is pulled medially. The transversalis fascia is opened and the epigastric vessels are identified: they are

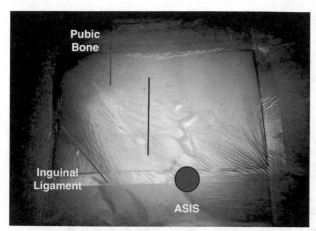

Fig. 6.1 Left inguinal region, landmarks in *red* (ASIS: anterior superior iliac spine) and incision line in *black*

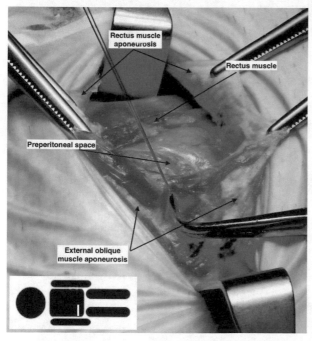

Fig. 6.2 Right inguinal region, the rectus muscle and the external oblique muscle aponeurosis are opened together and the fibers of the internal oblique and transversus muscle are split laterally. Here the ilioinguinal nerve has been found among the fibers of the internal oblique and transversus muscles and it is ready to be tied and cut

normally retracted medially and, if necessary, they are tied and cut safely [10]. Then, following the avascular plane just underlying the epigastric vessels, the preperitoneal space is approached (Fig. 6.3).

The blunt dissection proceeds laterally and cranially and the psoas muscle is detectable in a deep position [3, 10] with the genitofemoral nerve running over it. Cranial to the psoas muscle, lies the quadratum lumborum muscle where the ilioinguinal and iliohypogastric nerves run (Fig. 6.4). During the procedure for

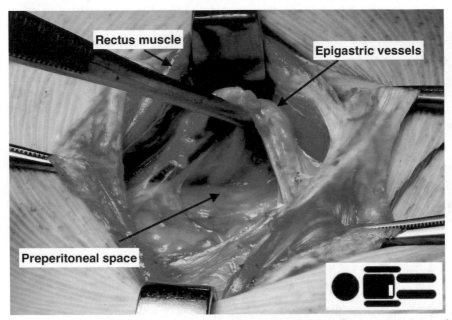

Fig. 6.3 Right inguinal region, a retractor pulls the rectus muscle medially, the epigastric vessels have been identified and the preperitoneal space is approached

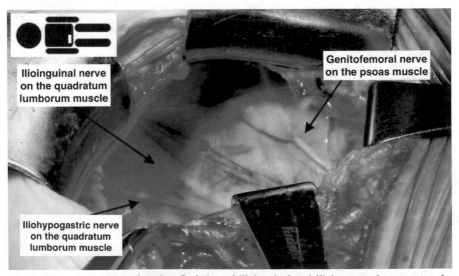

Fig. 6.4 Right preperitoneal region. Isolation of ilioinguinal and iliohypogastric nerves on the quadratum lumborum muscle and of the genitofemoral nerve on the psoas muscle

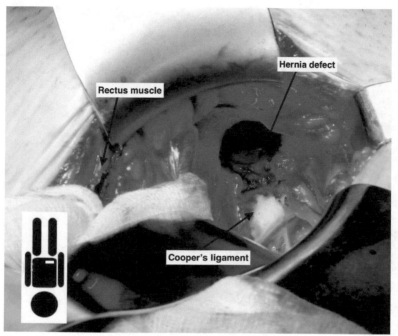

Fig. 6.5 Right preperitoneal region, isolation of the Cooper ligament and the hernia defect

the treatment of chronic postoperative pain, all the three nerves are tied, cut and buried (triple neurectomy) [9].

Proceeding with a blunt dissection at retropubic level, the Retzius space is reached and the Cooper's ligament is identified (Fig. 6.5) [3, 10]: scar tissue may be present after a prostatectomy or hysterectomy or radiotherapy and consequently urinary bladder dissection from the pubic symphysis may prove difficult. If the urinary bladder has been injured during this step, an absorbable suture is done and the urinary catheter is kept in place for one week after surgery.

Going from the pubic symphysis towards the psoas muscle, the Bogros space is approached and the external iliac vessels, the cord and the hernia sac, if present, are identified (Fig. 6.6) [3, 10].

If a plug has been placed during the previous surgery, scar adhesions will be present. This is the right time to remove a plug if the patient complains of chronic pain because it can be done safely and avoiding injury to nearby structures (iliac vein, bowel, vas, spermatic vessels, urinary bladder) (Fig. 6.7) [9]. Otherwise, if the aim of the surgery is to repair a recurrent hernia, the plug can be left in place if it does not interfere with the placement of the new mesh.

If a direct inguinal sac or a femoral sac is present, its reduction is possible with blunt traction movements and the transversalis fascia can be introflexed and fixed to the Cooper's ligament or rectus muscle (posterior face) so that the dead space is reduced, as is the risk of seroma formation [3, 10]. Then, the cord is surrounded by a path.

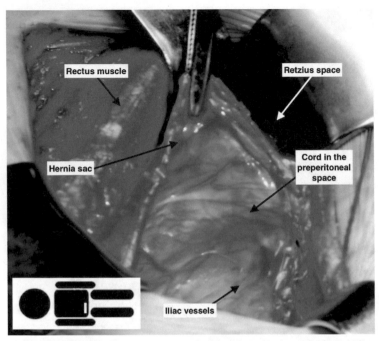

Fig. 6.6 Right preperitoneal region, the Bogros space is approached, an indirect inguinal sac is present, the cord is identified, the iliac vessels are covered by fat and lymphatic tissue

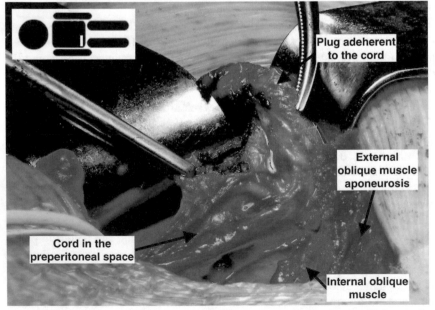

Fig. 6.7 Right preperitoneal region, isolation of the cord and of a plug previously placed adhering strictly to the vas and the cord. The plug will be removed

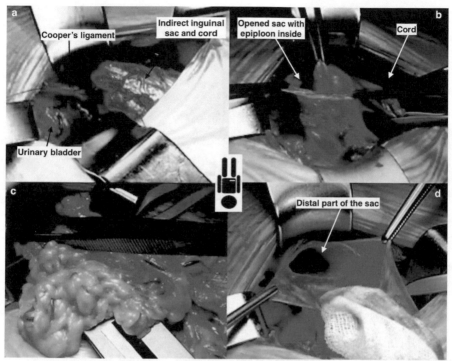

Fig. 6.8 Right preperitoneal region, isolation of incarcerated indirect recurrent hernia (**a**) with epiploon inside. The cord is surrounded by a blue path. The sac is opened (**b**) in order to complete the reduction of epiploon (**c**) in the abdominal cavity. A gauze is temporarily placed in the proximal part of the sac (**d**). The peritoneum will be closed and the distal part will be left in the scrotal cavity

In the case of an indirect inguinal hernia, the sac is found adherent to the spermatic cord and identification and division of one from the other is mandatory (Fig. 6.6). The inguinal sac is reduced with a gentle pulling movement from ahead to behind, in other words from the internal inguinal ring towards the preperitoneal space.

If a complete reduction of the sac is not possible (e.g., in the case of a huge inguinoscrotal or a multirecurrent hernia), opening of the sac is suggested (Fig.6.8) and, after the viscera have been reduced, the distal part of the sac is left and the peritoneum is closed with a running suture. If a real loss of substance is present, a vicryl or biological mesh is bridged to the peritoneum [3, 10]. In all cases, the cord or the round ligament is parietalized.

If the aim of the surgery is the treatment of postoperative pain, the next step is to remove the mesh placed during the previous surgery. Through the same incision, after dissection of the skin and subcutaneous space towards the pubic bone, the anterior region is approached, the external oblique aponeurosis is opened and the meshoma or mesh and suture or stitches can be completely removed (Fig. 6.9). It is important to remember that the cord may be found below the fascia but also

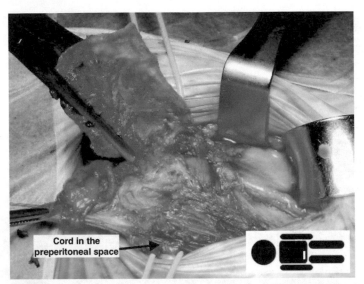

Fig. 6.9 The previously placed mesh is removed in the anterior inguinal region

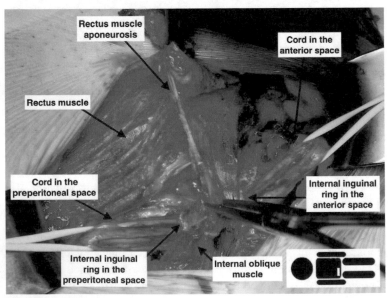

Fig. 6.10 Right inguinal region, after preperitoneal isolation of the cord (left side of the picture) through the same incision, the anterior inguinal region has been approached (right side of the picture), the previously place mesh has been removed, and the cord has been completely isolated

above the fascia, depending on the technique used in the previous surgery. So a prudent dissection is required to identify and preserve the cord (Fig. 6.10) [9].

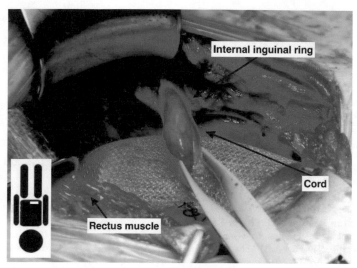

Fig. 6.11 Right preperitoneal region, a polypropylene mesh is placed, the cord passes through a hole in the prosthesis

The ilioinguinal and iliohypogastric nerves and the genital branch of the genitofemoral nerve can be sometimes re-identified and resected once again. This is not easy because of the scar tissue and adhesions due to previous surgery and the prosthesis previously placed. For this reason and to guarantee a complete triple neurectomy, the preperitoneal approach is necessary [9].

The next step is the placement of the mesh in the preperitoneal space: the original technique requires a polypropylene or polyester mesh, although we obtained excellent results also with a lightweight or biological absorbable mesh. The prosthesis has a rectangular shape with a length between 10 and 12 cm and a height between 14 and 15 cm, and it has a concavity along its bottom edge for the iliac vessels [3, 10].

The medial-inferior corner of the mesh is placed on the Cooper's ligament, the bottom edge along the iliac vessels and the lateral-inferior corner on the psoas muscle. Then the superior edge of the mesh is folded and placed underneath the rectus and oblique muscles, medially and laterally, respectively. The mesh is spread out and it covers and overlaps the entire myopectineal orifice.

The original technique has a sutureless mesh [3, 10], but during the learning curve and when a lightweight mesh is selected, a long-term absorbable or non-absorbable stitch can be placed on the Cooper's ligament and on the psoas muscle, paying attention to the nerves running along it [9, 10]. A second option could be glue fixation [9]. A modification of the technique can be a 5-6-cm right-angle incision on the superior edge, so that the cord or the round ligament can pass through, and then a runnning suture to close the mesh behind it (Fig. 6.11) [9]. The procedure is completed by closing the oblique muscle and rectus muscle aponeurosis.

References

1. Stoppa R, Petit J, Abourachid H (1972) Procédé original de plastie des hernies de l'aine: l'interposition sans fixation d'une prothèse en tulle de Dacron par voie médiane sous-péritonéale. Rev Med Picardie 1:46–48
2. Stoppa R, Petit J, Abourachid H et al (1973) Original procedure of groin hernia repair: interposition without fixation of Dacron tulle prosthesis by subperitoneal median approach. Chirurgie 99:119–123
3. Wantz GE (1989) Giant prosthetic reinforcement of the visceral sac. Surg Gynecol Obstet 169:408–417
4. Frauchaud H (1956) Anatomie chirurgicale des hernies de l'aine. Doin, Paris
5. Hair A, Duffy K, McLean Jet al (2000) Groin hernia repair in Scotland. Br J Surg 87:1722–1726
6. Cavalli M, Biondi A, Bruni PG, Campanelli G (2015) Giant inguinal hernia: the challenging hug technique. Hernia 19:775–783
7. Kurzer M, Belsham PA, Kark AE (2002) Prospective study of open preperitoneal mesh repair for recurrent inguinal hernia. Br J Surg 89:90–93
8. Campanelli G, Pettinari D, Nicolosi FM et al (2006) Inguinal hernia recurrence: classification and approach. Hernia 10:159–161
9. Campanelli G, Bertocchi V, Cavalli M et al (2013) Surgical treatment of chronic pain after inguinal hernia repair. Hernia 17:347–353
10. Olmi S, Erba L, Scaini A, Croce E (2006) Ernioplastica inguinale secondo Wantz. In: Olmi S, Croce E (eds) Chirurgia della parete addominale, 1st edn. Masson, Milano

Transinguinal Preperitoneal (TIPP) Repair

7

Frederik Christiaan Berrevoet

7.1 Introduction

The choice of a specific surgical technique to repair inguinal hernias depends on multiple factors such as the surgeon's preference, training, and capabilities and on logistical and socio-economical issues. In many countries, the Lichtenstein repair is still considered the gold standard for inguinal hernia repair. However, the increasing number of reports with high incidences of postoperative pain after open anterior mesh repair needs consideration [1–3]. The major factors responsible for both acute and chronic pain are the length of incision [4], nerve injury or entrapment, extensive dissection in the inguinal canal and fixation of the mesh with sutures or fixation devices [5]. To avoid especially neuropathic pain, of which the exact aetiology is still unknown, laparoscopic preperitoneal techniques have been described with the additional benefit of using intra-abdominal pressure to push the mesh against the underlying fascia as a more natural type of repair.

Due to the relatively long learning curve and some reports showing unacceptable high recurrence rates, during the last two decades open preperitoneal techniques have re-gained attention in the repair of inguinal hernias [6].

The traditional anterior approach is the most widely known and therefore reproducible by many surgeons. In transinguinal preperitoneal repair (TIPP), the preperitoneal space can be reached through the deep inguinal ring or through the medial inguinal defect by incising the transversalis fascia. This type of mesh repair is facilitated by the use of a memory-containing prosthesis. The memory ring offers, in contrast to some other techniques, an easy deployment of the patch in the preperitoneal space under good visualization of the groin structures. In this chapter we will give a detailed description of the TIPP technique that aims to provide a physiological type of repair, using only limited dissection in the inguinal canal with avoidance of the inguinal nerves and a short reconvalescence period.

F.C. Berrevoet (✉)
Department of General and Hepatopancreaticobiliairy Surgery and Liver Transplantation,
Ghent University Hospital and Medical School
Ghent, Belgium
e-mail: Frederik.berrevoet@ugent.be

G. Campanelli (Ed), *Inguinal Hernia Surgery,*
Updates in Surgery
DOI: 10.1007/978-88-470-3947-6_7, © Springer-Verlag Italia 2017

7.2   Surgical Technique

7.2.1   Indications and Contraindications

All patients, male and female, with a primary inguinal, femoral or obturator hernia are eligible for this technique. In cases of previous preperitoneal surgery, e.g., open prostatectomy with lymphadenectomy, bladder surgery and pelvic trauma surgery, or in cases of previous inguinal hernia surgery using the preperitoneal space for mesh location, the TIPP technique might succeed in only 50% of cases. In our experience, a prostatectomy with extensive lymphadenectomy seems to have a high conversion rate to a Lichtenstein repair. No other contraindications seem apparent.

7.2.2   Preoperative Preparation

For all techniques approaching the preperitoneal space, it is helpful and advantageous that the patient empties his/her bladder just prior to surgery. This way, mobilization of the lateral and ventral wall of the bladder will be facilitated and no Foley catheter is needed.

7.2.3   Anaesthesia

The procedure can be performed under local anaesthesia (with sedation) or using spinal anaesthesia. Straining and coughing might help to spread the mesh and enable the surgeon to check the correct position of the mesh at the end of the procedure. Because manipulation of the peritoneum during dissection can lead to additional stress and pain, it might be more troublesome to use local anaesthesia in younger patients as they are generally more anxious during surgery. Spinal anaesthesia, using ropivacaine 0.2% without admixture of opioids does not induce unacceptably high urinary retention rates leading to unplanned admissions. An additional local incisional block with ropivacaine 0.2% can be very useful, especially in day-care treatment. In other situations general anaesthesia might be the option of choice.

7.2.4   Incision

After disinfection and sterile draping of the groin area, the operation starts by drawing a line between the lower edge of the superior anterior iliac spine and the pubic tubercle. The distance is then measured. For most patients this will range between 10 and 13 cm. Halfway along this line we start the incision and proceed medially for 3 cm at an angle of approximately 30 degrees (Fig. 7.1). By doing

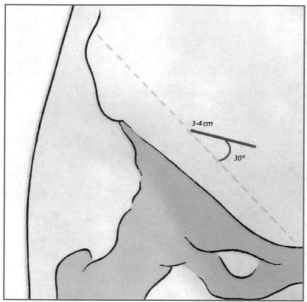

Fig. 7.1 Skin incision for a right inguinal hernia starting halfway along the line between the superior anterior iliac spine and the pubic tubercle over 3 cm to the medial side

so, we centre the incision precisely over the deep inguinal ring and the epigastric vessels. The iliac vessels will then always be just at the lateral edge of the incision and serve as an important reference point at the time of mesh introduction.

7.2.5 Superficial Dissection

The skin, subcutaneous fat, and Scarpa's fascia are opened down to the aponeurosis of the external oblique muscle and the external orifice can be visualized. The external oblique aponeurosis is then opened, taking caution not to harm the ilioinguinal nerve, and the inguinal canal is exposed (Fig. 7.2).

An important modification compared to the former description of this technique [7] is *not* to perform extensive dissection to locate the hernia defect, but, if possible, to let the patient strain or cough and in that way visualize the defect. There is absolutely no reason to completely section the cremasteric muscle and to skeletonise the cord structures. This may only increase the harm done to the inguinal nerves.

7.2.6 Approach for Indirect Hernias (Fig. 7.3)

In the case of an indirect hernia, the sac is completely dissected until its entrance through the internal orifice. At the level of the orifice, the preperitoneal fat can

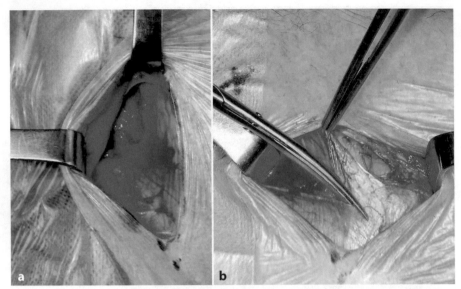

Fig. 7.2 a Superficial dissection of the subcutaneous fat and Scarpa's fascia. **b** Incision of the aponeurosis of the external oblique muscle

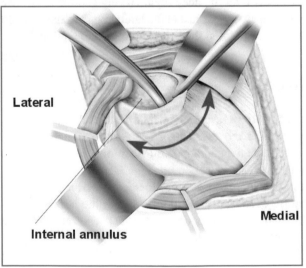

Fig. 7.3 The approach for entering the preperitoneal space in case of an indirect hernia

Lateral

Medial

Internal annulus

now be seen. It is important at this time to visualize the epigastric vessels before entering the preperitoneal space. The posterior sheet of the transversalis fascia should be opened at the level of the dilated deep internal ring to enter the space

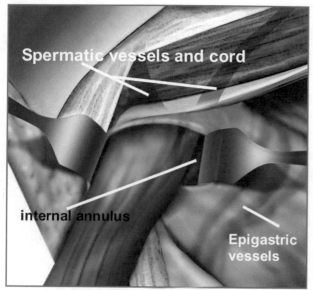

Fig. 7.4 Complete parietalization of the cord structures

of Bogros. From that moment on, the epigastric vessels will be retracted softly upwards. After palpation of both Cooper's ligament and the pubic bone to ensure the dissection will be done in the right avascular preperitoneal plane, gauze can be introduced into the preperitoneal space towards the space of Retzius. By doing so, most of the dissection medially will be performed bluntly. The index finger can now be introduced medially performing further dissection, first cranially, leaving the preperitoneal fat attached to the peritoneum. The fatty tissue is then swept off from the iliopubic branch of the iliac bone, the pubic symphysis, the rectus muscle and the transverse muscle in succession, thus enlarging the preperitoneal space to accommodate the mesh.

The next step, crucial for a good accommodation of the mesh in the preperitoneal pocket, is to parietalize the peritoneum off the cord structures as far as possible, even inside the abdominal cavity where the spermatic cord separates from the spermatic vessels (Fig. 7.4). In very obese patients this can be difficult to achieve through a 3 cm incision. However, especially for larger indirect hernias this is essential for preventing later recurrences. By doing this there is no need to create a new internal orifice.

A last critical point in using this technique is to obtain a sufficient pocket at the lateral side of the internal orifice. To facilitate this part of the dissection, it can sometimes be helpful to introduce gauze laterally. One should only be satisfied with the created pocket once the index finger can reach the superior anterior iliac spine easily.

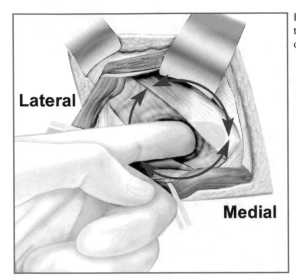

Fig. 7.5 The approach for entering the preperitoneal space in the case of a direct hernia defect

7.2.7   Approach for Direct or Femoral Hernias (Fig. 7.5)

In case the surgeon feels more comfortable to completely dissect the direct hernia sac, in the absence of an indirect component, he can incise the direct hernia sac (both layers of the transversalis fascia have to be incised) at its base circumferentially. The preperitoneal fat will then immediately be visualized and you can enter the preperitoneal space. Again, the epigastric vessels should be identified, on the lateral side of the defect in this situation, and protected by a retractor upwards. The preperitoneal space is created in the same manner as in the indirect hernia. In cases of a femoral or obturator hernia, the transversalis fascia has to be incised from the internal ring.

In our experience, we prefer handling all types of hernia through the deep internal ring as it is very easy to reduce direct hernias by approaching these from the lateral side, while reduction and dissection of an indirect hernia sac might be more difficult. In the case of a combination of an indirect and direct hernia, or when the direct component is difficult to reduce, one could also prefer to open the transversalis fascia over a few centimetres through the deep inguinal ring.

7.2.8   Introduction of the Mesh and Adequate Mesh Placement

After creation of the appropriate pocket, a malleable flat retractor is introduced medially to recline peritoneum, preperitoneal fat and the lateral aspect of the bladder. Introduction of the mesh can now be performed, by sliding the mesh over the malleable retractor.

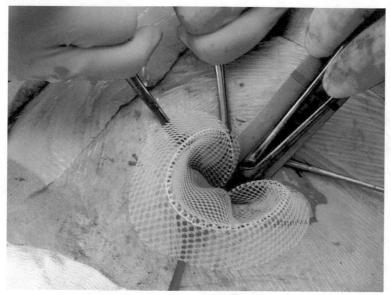

Fig. 7.6 Introduction of the mesh by sliding it over the retractor

The use of a mesh with a memory facilitates the introduction and fast placement. Different meshes are available. The Polysoft mesh consists of a polypropylene mesh with a resorbable memory ring. It has an oval shape and exists in two sizes: medium (14 × 7.5 cm) and large (16 × 9.5 cm). Laterally, a notch has been manufactured in the mesh to allow proper deployment over the iliac vessels. The main disadvantage of this mesh is the interrupted memory at the lateral side, which limits the complete deployment of the mesh in some cases, which might lead to pain or long-term recurrences.

Another possible mesh frame is the Rebound HRD shield, which consists of a large polypropylene mesh with a non-resorbable nitinol frame. It is also available in two sizes: small (14.93 × 10.31 cm) and large (16 × 11 cm). This mesh has a continuous memory ring that facilitates lateral flat mesh placement.

The medial side of the mesh is grasped with a blunt clamp, and the mesh is introduced in the direction of the pubis, up to the tendon of the rectus muscle, keeping the malleable retractor still in place (Fig 7.6). The clamp can then be removed from the mesh as well as the malleable retractor. Although the created pocket is medially large enough to do so, it is important not to introduce the mesh too medially. Especially for indirect hernias, an adequate overlap of the mesh lateral to the deep internal ring is necessary.

From that point the mesh has to be manipulated by two forceps at its edges to allow perfect placement both underneath the muscles and laterally covering the iliac vessels until the outer tip of the prosthesis almost reaches the superior anterior iliac spine. By placing a retractor in the lateral pocket and keeping it up, this aspect of the technique can be facilitated.

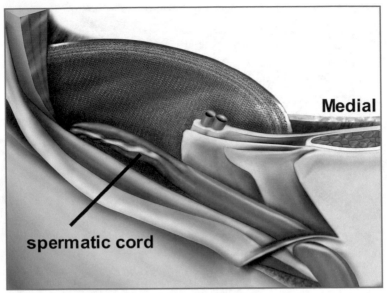

Fig. 7.7 Final position of the mesh covering all orifices

7.2.9   Final Position of the Patch (Fig. 7.7)

Further accommodation of the mesh can be achieved by a Valsalva manoeuvre, by increasing the pulmonary end-expiratory pressure by the anaesthesiologist, or by letting the patient strain and cough in the case of local or spinal anaesthesia. Once the mesh seems to be in position, it is important to check medially that there is sufficient overlap of the pubic tubercle and on the lateral side that there is flat mesh deployment towards the iliac spine.

7.2.10   Fixation and Closure

No suturing or tacks are necessary to fix this type of mesh. The memory ring will hold tension on the mesh and as the created preperitoneal pocket just matches the size of the mesh to be used, migration of the mesh seems impossible. The aponeurosis of the external oblique muscle is then closed using resorbable sutures 3/0. Subcutaneous tissue and skin are closed as well with absorbable sutures 2/0 and 4/0, respectively.

7.2.11   Postoperative Recommendations

In total this procedure takes between 15 and 45 minutes depending on the size of the hernia and the dissection necessary to completely free the sac. We advise patients to take analgesics for 2 days and mobilize from day 1 without limitations. The time patients need to return to their normal daily activity is between 2 and 4 days and the time to return to full activity, including their job and sports, is around 14 days.

7.3   Discussion

In our opinion, five issues need to be addressed when evaluating possible aetiologies for pain after inguinal hernia repair: small incision; minimal dissection around the inguinal nerves; location of the mesh in the preperitoneal space, and not in contact with the nerves; minimal or no fixation of the mesh; no extensive amount of material, to prevent severe local inflammation and fibrosis around the nerves and the cord structures during tissue ingrowth.

The avascular preperitoneal space is biomechanically and physiologically an ideal location for our mesh reinforcement, as it is avascular and during ingrowth no scar tissue will implicate the nerves or the cord in the long term.

Using an incision of only 3 cm is beneficial for the patient, considering both aesthetics and postoperative pain. Although perhaps not important to surgeons ("the greater the incision, the greater the surgeon"), patients tend to compare the aesthetic aspects of surgery, certainly in competition with laparoscopic techniques.

Although this transinguinal approach still includes dissection around the inguinal nerves, we advocate minimal dissection around the hernia sac only and not to take down all cremasteric muscles, nor to free all boundaries of the inguinal canal itself as in a Lichtenstein repair. Checking for indirect hernias in the case of medial defects is of course mandatory to prevent early recurrences.

To allow quick and adequate placement of a mesh through this limited incision in the preperitoneal space, a mesh with enough memory is advisable. Moreover, although the transinguinal preperitoneal approach itself is far from innovative [7–11], this technique allows for an efficient repair with adequate visualization of inguinal anatomy, which is rather difficult using a flat mesh.

Fixation is one of the main aetiologies for postoperative pain in all mesh augmentations for abdominal wall surgery. Therefore, we consider it favourable, as in laparoscopic inguinal hernia repair, that this mesh needs no or minimal fixation. The intra-abdominal pressure as well as the forces of the abdominal muscles will keep the mesh in place. Compared to the Lichtenstein method or the plug-and-patch techniques, this might most probably decrease the amount of postoperative pain.

There is absolutely no need to create a new internal orifice by splitting the mesh. This implicates, however, and this needs to be stressed, a complete parietalization of the cord up to the level where the vessels separate from the spermatic cord "intra-abdominally". The same idea is true for laparoscopic techniques, where the mesh is never split. To deal with possible shortcomings on the lateral border of the patch, large-sized patches are appropriate for most indirect hernias.

The TIPP technique is a preperitoneal mesh repair that can be offered to patients using a highly standardized surgical technique. In the case of adequate knowledge of the preperitoneal anatomy the TIPP technique is easy to perform and, according to the current literature, it is efficient, safe and with a low rate of chronic pain [12–15].

References

1. Aasvang EK, Bay-Nielsen M, Kehlet H (2006) Pain and functional impairment 6 years after inguinal herniorrhaphy. Hernia 10:316–321
2. Bay-Nielsen M, Nilsson E, Nordin P et al (2004) Chronic pain after open mesh and sutured repair of indirect inguinal hernia in young males. Br J Surg 91:1372–1376
3. Callesen T, Bech K, Kehlet H (1999) Prospective study of chronic pain after groin hernia repair. Br J Surg 86:1528–1531
4. Champault G, Bernard C, Rizk N et al (2007) Inguinal hernia repair: the choice of prosthesis outweighs that of technique. Hernia 11:125–128
5. Franneby U, Sandblom G, Nordin P et al (2006) Risk factors for long-term pain after hernia surgery. Ann Surg 244:212–219
6. Neumayer L, Giobbie-Hurder A, Jonasson O et al (2004) Open mesh versus laparoscopic mesh repair of inguinal hernia. N Engl J Med 350:1819–1827
7. Muldoon RL, Marchant K, Johnson DD et al (2004) Lichtenstein vs anterior preperitoneal prosthetic mesh placement in open inguinal hernia repair: a prospective, randomized trial. Hernia 8:98–103
8. Stoppa R, Petit J, Abourachid H et al (1973) Original procedure of groin hernia repair: interposition without fixation of Dacron tulle prosthesis by subperitoneal median approach. Chirurgie 99:119–123 [Article in French]
9. Rives J, Lardennois B, Flament JB et al (1973) The Dacron mesh sheet, treatment of choice of inguinal hernias in adults. Apropos of 183 cases. Chirurgie 99:564–575 [Article in French]
10. Arlt G, Schumpelick V (1997) Transinguinal preperitoneal mesh-plasty (TIPP) in management of recurrent inguinal hernia. Chirurg 68:1235–1238 [Article in German]
11. Awad SS, Yallampalli S, Srour AM et al (2007) Improved outcomes with the Prolene Hernia System mesh compared with the time-honored Lichtenstein onlay mesh repair for inguinal hernia repair. Am J Surg 193:697–701
12. Berrevoet F, Sommeling C, De Gendt S et al (2009) The preperitoneal memory-ring patch for inguinal hernia: a prospective multicentric feasibility study. Hernia 13:243–249
13. Berrevoet F, Maes L, Reyntjens K et al (2010) Transinguinal preperitoneal memory ring patch versus Lichtenstein repair for unilateral inguinal hernias. Langenbecks Arch Surg 395:557–562
14. Berrevoet F, Vanlander A, Bontinck J et al (2013) Open preperitoneal mesh repair of inguinal hernias using a mesh with nitinol memory frame. Hernia 17:365–371
15. Koning GG, Keus F, Koeslag L et al (2012) Randomized clinical trial of chronic pain after the transinguinal preperitoneal technique compared with Lichtenstein's method for inguinal hernia repair. Br J Surg 99:1365–1373

Open New Simplified Totally Extraperitoneal (ONSTEP) Technique for Inguinal Hernia Repair

8

Jacob Rosenberg and Kristoffer Andresen

8.1 Introduction

The ONSTEP technique for inguinal hernia repair was developed by two surgeons from Portugal, Lorenzo and da Costa [1]. For several years there has been a trend towards placing the mesh in the preperitoneal space rather than below the external aponeurosis as in the Lichtenstein repair. The reason for this has been reports of reduced pain after surgery, especially levels of chronic pain, with the preperitoneal mesh replacement as in laparoscopic repair [2].

There are several different operative techniques available for preperitoneal mesh replacement including the transinguinal preperitoneal approach (TIPP) [3] and transrectus sheath extraperitoneal procedure (TREPP) [4] and others, but these techniques may be difficult to approach for the novice surgeon. Thus, Lorenzo and da Costa thought that there was a need for a new method with a technically easier approach and therefore a shorter learning curve for the young surgeons.

The present status for the ONSTEP technique is that it is currently used in several surgical departments and there are also a few ongoing research projects evaluating the technique [5, 6]. Currently, the technique has only been spread to some countries in Europe, mainly because the mesh has not been available in the United States until recently. Surgeons in the United States and Asia will soon be exposed to this new technique, hopefully resulting in more scientific trials evaluating the pros and cons.

The aim of the present chapter is to introduce the ONSTEP technique and give an overview of the current available clinical data. Furthermore, we discuss the technique's perspectives and the possible future role of ONSTEP in inguinal hernia repair in adults.

J. Rosenberg (✉)
Department of Surgery, Herlev Hospital
Herlev, Denmark
e-mail: jacob.rosenberg@regionh.dk

G. Campanelli (Ed), *Inguinal Hernia Surgery,*
Updates in Surgery
DOI: 10.1007/978-88-470-3947-6_8, © Springer-Verlag Italia 2017

8.2   The ONSTEP Technique

The ONSTEP technique is special because it involves both the preperitoneal space
as well as the space between the external and internal aponeurosis. Thus, it can be
seen as a mixture of a preperitoneal technique and a fully external approach [1].
Because of space limitations the reader is kindly referred to a detailed description
of the operative technique published previously [1].

8.2.1   Why a Technique that Involves two Different Planes?

An intriguing part of this surgical technique is that it involves two different
planes. The medial part of the mesh is placed in the preperitoneal space, the space
of Retzius, and the lateral part of the mesh is placed between the internal and
external aponeurosis, i.e. the same place as we place the mesh in the conventional
Lichtenstein repair. The mesh is not sutured to tissue and this special mesh
placement will ensure that it stays in place even though it is not fixated to the body
structures. This special mesh placement also has the special effect that it will grab
the abdominal wall, especially when the patient is standing up where gravity will
put force on a flat mesh placed simultaneously between the external and internal
aponeurosis (lateral part) as well as a mesh placed in the preperitoneal space
(medial part). In the ONSTEP technique the mesh has a kind of a handgrip shape
holding the abdominal wall and thereby keeping the hernias in place. This may
be the mechanism of action of the ONSTEP technique and could explain the low
recurrence rates and together with the lack of mesh fixation and the very gentle
dissection technique, probably explain the extremely low risk of chronic pain [7].

8.2.2   The Onflex Mesh

A special mesh has been designed for the ONSTEP operation (Fig. 8.1). This mesh
is called the Onflex mesh. It has a stiff ring along the border of the mesh in order
to keep it deployed in the preperitoneal space. The ring is made of absorbable
material so that it will not cause concern for the patient. Before the Onflex mesh
was available we used the Polysoft mesh for the ONSTEP operation. This mesh
has a non-absorbable ring, so that skinny patients could sometimes feel it and had
pain from especially the lateral part of the mesh which lies between the external
and internal oblique aponeurosis. If the patient is skinny and has the Onflex mesh
in the correct position, then even though he or she may feel the lateral part of the
ring in the beginning, these complaints will disappear when the ring is absorbed.
The mesh is made of polypropylene, is low weight and with large pore sizes.
This should enable better ingrowth in the healing period after mesh placement.
Furthermore, it has a pocket which will make it easier to position the mesh in
the preperitoneal space. When the mesh is positioned the pocket is meant for the
index finger of the surgeon.

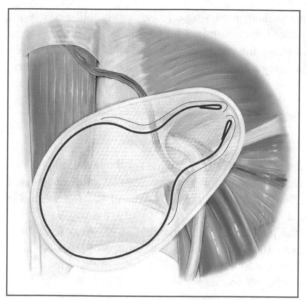

Fig. 8.1 The Onflex mesh for ONSTEP inguinal hernia repair. Reproduced with permission from Bard-Davol Inc.

8.2.3   Pain from the Recoil Ring

There are thousands of patients who have had the ONSTEP procedure with the Polysoft mesh. In the Polysoft mesh the ring is non-absorbable and if the patient is skinny, there may be complaints from the lateral part of the mesh where the ring will lie close to the skin. In such a case we usually recommend that the patients should wait for 6 months in order for the mesh to be fully integrated into the tissue, especially in the preperitoneal position and on the muscle plate between the two aponeuroses. Then the patient is offered a small reoperation where an incision of about 1 cm is performed on top of the palpable part of the ring corresponding to the lateral part of the mesh. Then the two ends of the ring are dissected and cut and the ring can be withdrawn in full. We have made a video clip of this procedure [8]. Usually after ring removal the patient will have no complaints.

8.2.4   Recurrence Repair after Previous ONSTEP

Some surgeons may have concern about how to repair a recurrence after previous ONSTEP repair, because the mesh will be present both preperitoneally as well as between the two aponeuroses laterally. It is, however, no problem at all to do a recurrence repair after a previous ONSTEP. It may preferably be done by two different approaches, one being a simple re-ONSTEP procedure, and the other by laparoscopic operation. If doing a re-ONSTEP then you dissect on top of the previously placed mesh, with dissection between the mesh and the pubic bone making a new space for a new Onflex mesh. A mesh is then placed between the old mesh and the pubic bone without removing any part of the old mesh. With a laparoscopic repair we use the transabdominal preperitoneal (TAPP) approach and it has been easy to take down the peritoneum from inside and then simply put a standard flat mesh in the preperitoneal space as a standard TAPP procedure.

8.3   Clinical Data

The first clinical data regarding the ONSTEP technique is a large and impressive series of patients from two centers. The inventors presented 693 patients operated with the technique and followed up for one year [1]. Several findings from this paper showed a promise of a better open technique. Firstly, the degree of pain was very low, and none of the patients had chronic pain at one-year follow-up. Secondly, only four recurrences (0.6%) were found with three of them being in women. This has led the inventors to slightly modify the technique for female patients. Third, a very short duration of surgery – mean (SD): 17 (6) minutes – was found, which can be cost-saving for a department since it will allow for more patients being operated in one day. Such a large series with promising results called for further scientific exploration of the technique and also justified the conduction of randomized controlled trials. Surgeons from other countries in Europe visited the inventors, learned the technique, and started operating at their own centers.

The first published results from outside Portugal were from Denmark and included 80 patients, with follow-up by standardized questionnaires [9]. Results were good, albeit with the use of questionnaires and not a dichotomous pain registration some patients were found to have pain, but at very low levels. Later, results were presented from a series from Greece [10]. Results were still similar, with low levels of postoperative pain and no patients with chronic pain. A similar report was published from the Czech Republic [11], still with promising results (Table 8.1).

The non-controlled series outside the departments of the inventors supported the promising results, but are all at risk of bias since no randomization and/or control group was added to any of the studies. Furthermore, follow-up time and methods were not standardized. Therefore, there was a need for randomized clinical trials. As of December 2015, two prospective trials can be found on the WHO trial search portal [12]. Both studies are from Denmark. One is the ONSTEP versus Lichtenstein (ONLi) study, with 290 included patients and one-year follow-up [5]. The other, ONSTEP versus Laparoscopy (ONLap), is still recruiting patients [13]. Both studies are being conducted as multicenter studies with general surgical departments, i.e. not specialized hernia centers.

The early results from the ONLi trial demonstrated a safe implementation of the technique, with results similar to the Lichtenstein technique [13]. The only significant difference found in the early results was the duration of surgery. Patients were followed up with several questionnaires and at 6-month follow-up a significant difference was found, favoring the ONSTEP technique in the number

Table 8.1 Case series

Country	No	Study type	Persistent Pain	Recurrence	Minutes
Portugal [1]	693	Case series	0%	4 (0.6)	17 (+6)
Denmark [9]	80	Case series	4.5%	0	24 (13-53)
Greece [10]	33	Case series	0%	0	33.28 (+11.69)
Czech [11]	72+25	Case series	0%	2	18-35

of patients experiencing pain during sexual activity [14]. Follow-up for pain at 6 and 12 months showed that the number of patients with non-sexual pain as well as the intensity of pain were similar in the two groups. A noteworthy finding was that two patients in the Lichtenstein group experienced disabling chronic pain after surgery. Both had the mesh surgically removed as well as neurectomy conducted around 6 months postoperatively with complete resolving of pain for one patient but persisting pain for the other. No patients in the ONSTEP group experienced these disabling symptoms.

The ONLap study is designed to show non-inferiority between the ONSTEP and the laparoscopic technique (TAPP), i.e. similar levels of postoperative pain. The rationale is that the ONSTEP technique has some advantages compared to laparoscopy and therefore if non-inferiority can be demonstrated regarding pain other advantages will justify it as a valid alternative. The advantages are that the ONSTEP technique has a shorter duration of surgery, it does not require the same expensive equipment as laparoscopic repair, and it is likely to have a much shorter learning curve.

8.4 Learning, Training, and Implementation

The ONSTEP procedure has a shorter duration of surgery than a standard Lichtenstein or laparoscopic repair and surgeons learning the technique find it easy to learn. To our knowledge, it has primarily been learned by surgeons already familiar with hernia repair, and therefore experience is lacking as to how well younger surgeons in training can pick up the technique. We believe that it will be easier to learn than the Lichtenstein repair, but solid data are missing to support this. It is very likely easier to learn the ONSTEP technique compared to the laparoscopic techniques (TEP or TAPP), since no endoscopic skills are needed.

Implementation of the ONSTEP technique can be done if surgeons with experience are willing to learn the technique. It has been suggested that the optimal way of learning the technique and subsequent implementation is when the training is done as proctoring [15]. When training surgeons in the ONSTEP technique, some concerns and difficulties need to be addressed, such as fear of the preperitoneal space [16].

8.5   Health Economics

A formal health economics analysis comparing the ONSTEP method with laparoscopic and Lichtenstein repair has not been conducted yet, but it is planned to use the data from the ONLi and ONLap randomized trials [5, 13] for such an analysis. It is expected that the ONSTEP method will prove to be cost-saving compared to the laparoscopic techniques and comparable or maybe even cost-saving compared to the Lichtenstein technique.

Compared to the laparoscopic technique, the Lichtenstein technique has been demonstrated to result in lower costs [17], mainly due to the cost of equipment, sterilization, and time in the operating room. The level of pain, minor complications and sick-leave is expected to be similar between the laparoscopic and the ONSTEP technique, so the cost from sick leave will probably be equal in the two groups. The laparoscopic technique results in a low, albeit increased risk of serious complications that can result in increased costs.

Compared to Lichtenstein, the costs of conducting the ONSTEP are more or less comparable but with a more expensive mesh. However, the price of the mesh might be justified by the shorter duration of surgery, which in some healthcare systems is an important economic factor. However, it is well known that the Lichtenstein technique carries a risk of serious disabling chronic pain, that results in tremendous cost for society because of resulting unemployment, for the employer because of long sick leave and for the insurance, be it public or private, because of unemployment benefits. The development of disabling chronic pain seems so far to be avoided with the use of the ONSTEP technique.

Furthermore, if the assumptions regarding a shorter learning curve are true, younger surgeons will not need the same amount of supervision, which can free hands in the surgical department and thereby be cost-saving, compared to training surgeons for the Lichtenstein or laparoscopic repairs.

Firm conclusions regarding the health economics aspect of the ONSTEP technique can only be made when results from the ongoing trials are combined and analyzed.

8.6   Perspectives

If data with the ONSTEP procedure continue to be robust and shown by different research groups to produce distinctly low levels of severe disabling chronic pain and comparable levels of acute pain and recurrences, then there may be a place for the ONSTEP procedure in the routine surgical armamentarium for repair of inguinal hernias. The procedure is fast and easy to learn, as well as advantageous compared with both the Lichtenstein and the laparoscopic procedure. Thus, ONSTEP may be first choice for primary inguinal hernias in men. In women it may be different since the operative procedure is different and technically more difficult than in men.

Table 8.2 Suggested treatment strategies of inguinal hernias. This could become effective if other research groups can reproduce the findings and the health economics analysis supports use of the Onstep technique

Current hernia	Previous operation	Recommended procedure
Male primary hernia	–	Onstep
Male, recurrent hernia	Lichtenstein Laparoscopic repair Onstep	Laparoscopic repair Onstep Laparoscopic repair or Onstep
Female, primary hernia	–	Laparoscopic repair
Female, recurrent hernia	Open procedure Laparoscopic repair	Laparoscopic repair Lichtenstein
Male, special cases (prostate cancer, extensive surgery, etc.)	–	Onstep or Lichtenstein

It could therefore be argued, that the laparoscopic procedure should still be first choice for women, as recommended in previous guidelines [18, 19].

If the patient has a recurrent hernia then an ONSTEP procedure may be used after previous ONSTEP or after previous laparoscopic repair. If the patient has a previous Lichtenstein repair, then a laparoscopic approach will probably be the easiest technically to perform. The main goal of changing strategy for choice of operation for inguinal hernia repair will be to avoid the Lichtenstein procedure because of the well-known production of severe disabling chronic pain in some patients. A new strategy could therefore be as shown in Table 8.2. This, however, has to be supported by trial data from other research groups confirming the current available results, as well as a health economics analysis showing advantages for the ONSTEP procedure compared to the Lichtenstein as well the laparoscopic approach.

8.7 Conclusions

The ONSTEP procedure was introduced by two surgeons from Portugal and has been used in the inventors' clinics with great success. It thereafter spread to several European countries by proctoring initially at the clinic in Porto and after that also through local training in other countries. Randomized trials have been performed and until now they have shown advantages for the ONSTEP procedure compared with Lichtenstein regarding sexual dysfunction after operation. Another very interesting feature of the ONSTEP procedure is that until now, after thousands of procedures, not a single patient with severe disabling chronic pain has been produced. This is in contrast to the Lichtenstein procedure where it is well known that some patients will develop severe disabling chronic pain. Overall, the ONSTEP procedure seems to be very promising and will probably find its place in routine inguinal hernia repair in the near future.

References

1. Lourenço A, da Costa RS (2013) The ONSTEP inguinal hernia repair technique: initial clinical experience of 693 patients, in two institutions. Hernia 17:357–364
2. Sevonius D, Montgomery A, Smedberg S, Sandblom G (2016) Chronic groin pain, discomfort and physical disability after recurrent groin hernia repair: impact of anterior and posterior mesh repair. Hernia 20:43–53
3. Pélissier EP, Ngo P, Gayet B (2011) Transinguinal preperitoneal patch (TIPP) under local anesthesia with sedation. Am Surg 77:1681–1684
4. Lange JF, Lange MM, Voropai DA et al (2014) Trans rectus sheath extra-peritoneal procedure (TREPP) for inguinal hernia: the first 1,000 patients. World J Surg 38:1922–1928
5. Andresen K, Burcharth J, Rosenberg J (2013) Lichtenstein versus Onstep for inguinal hernia repair: protocol for a double-blinded randomised trial. Dan Med J 60:A4729
6. Andresen K, Burcharth J, Rosenberg J (2015) Onstep versus laparoscopy for inguinal hernia repair. A protocol for a randomized clinical trial. Dan Med J 62:A5169
7. Öberg S, Andresen K, Hauge D, Rosenberg J (2016) Recurrence mechanisms after inguinal hernia repair by the Onstep technique – a case series. Hernia, in press
8. Öberg S, Andresen K, Rosenberg J (2016) How to surgically remove the permanent mesh ring after the Onstep procedure for alleviation of chronic pain following inguinal hernia repair. Case Reports in Surgery, article ID 5209095
9. Andresen K, Burcharth J, Rosenberg J (2015) The initial experience of introducing the Onstep technique for inguinal hernia repair in a general surgical department. Scand J Surg 104:61–65
10. Marinis A, Psimitis I (2014) The open new simplified totally extra-peritoneal (ONSTEP) inguinal hernia repair: initial experience with a novel technique. Hell Cheirourgike 86:362–367
11. Kohoutek L, Musil J, Plecháčová P, Gryga A (2015) Operace tříselné kýly technikou ONTEP [The ONSTEP inguinal hernia repair technique]. Rozhl Chir 94:152–155
12. World Health Organization. International Clinical Trials Registry Platform. http://apps.who.int/trialsearch. 21 December, 2015
13. Andresen K, Burcharth J, Fonnes S et al (2015) Short-term outcome after Onstep versus Lichtenstein technique for inguinal hernia repair: results from a randomized clinical trial. Hernia 19:871–877
14. Andresen K, Burcharth J, Fonnes S et al (2016) Sexual dysfunction after inguinal hernia repair with Onstep versus Lichtenstein technique: a randomized clinical trial. Hernia, in press
15. Rosenberg J, Andresen K, Laursen J (2014) Team training (training at own facility) versus individual surgeon's training (training at trainer's facility) when implementing a new surgical technique: example from the ONSTEP inguinal hernia repair. Surg Res Pract 2014:762761
16. Andresen K, Laursen J, Rosenberg J (2016) Difficulties and problematic steps in teaching the Onstep technique for inguinal hernia repair – results from a focus group interview. Surg Res Pract 2016: 4787648
17. Medical Research Council Laparoscopic Groin Hernia Trial Group (2001) Cost-utility analysis of open versus laparoscopic groin hernia repair: results from a multicentre randomized clinical trial. Br J Surg 88:653–661
18. Rosenberg J, Bisgaard T, Kehlet H et al (2011) Danish Hernia Database recommendations for the management of inguinal and femoral hernia in adults. Dan Med Bull 58:C4243
19. Miserez M, Peeters E, Aufenacker T et al (2014) Update with level 1 studies of the European Hernia Society guidelines on the treatment of inguinal hernia in adult patients. Hernia 18:151–163

Polysoft Patch for Inguinal Hernia Repair

9

Edouard P. Pélissier, Giel G. Koning, and Philippe Ngo

9.1. Introduction

The Polysoft patch for inguinal hernia repair was conceived on the basis of the following specifications:

- preperitoneal repair by a minimally invasive inguinal approach
- introduction and deployment of a prosthetic patch through the hernia orifice, without any other damage to the abdominal wall
- covering of the weak inguinal area and femoral orifice with minimal overlapping on visceral and vascular structures
- limiting the amount of foreign material to one single mesh layer.
- sutureless technique.

A flat mesh, equipped with a memory-ring made of absorbable material, so that only the flat mesh remained in place after the memory-ring was absorbed, fulfilled these specifications. This was the concept of the initial Pélissier patent (1998).

Two trials were undertaken by the inventing author to assess this concept. The first one was carried out on a series of patients with a weak posterior wall, using a technique derived from the Rives technique, which consisted of preperitoneal placement of a patch covering only the weak inguinal area and trying to reduce fixation [1]. Nevertheless, in most cases sutures could not be avoided, due to the flexibility of the mesh. Consequently, a new trial was carried out, using a flat mesh equipped with a sort of memory-ring made with a PDS cord [2]. Though it was not an actual recoil ring, deployment of the patch was facilitated and fixation sutures were reduced to a minimum.

Later on, collaboration with Davol (a subsidiary of Bard Inc.) to develop this concept resulted in the Polysoft patch. Despite the initial specifications, for technical reasons the patch was not equipped with an absorbable memory-ring, but with a ring made of flexible polyethylene. In the first feasibility study of Polysoft,

E.P. Pélissier (✉)
The Hernia Institute Paris
Paris, France
e-mail: pelissier.edouard@wanadoo.fr

G. Campanelli (Ed), *Inguinal Hernia Surgery,*
Updates in Surgery
DOI: 10.1007/978-88-470-3947-6_9, © Springer-Verlag Italia 2017

in two-thirds of indirect hernias the patch was split to accommodate the spermatic cord, in accordance with the Rives technique, and in one-third of the cases the cord was parietalized and the patch was not split [3]. Two recurrences protruding through the slit in the patch occurred in the first 171 cases [4]. Considering this fact and the experience of Berrevoet et al. [5], who immediately started parietalizing the cord instead of splitting the patch, the inventing author definitively switched to parietalizing the cord and not splitting the patch [6].

9.2   The TIPP (Transinguinal Preperitoneal Patch) Technique

9.2.1   Operative Technique

A short (3-5 cm) skin incision is carried out at the level of the deep inguinal orifice. The external oblique aponeurosis is incised and a self-retaining retractor (e.g., Gelpi) is placed. The ilioinguinal nerve is identified and preserved; identification of the iliohypogastric nerve and genital branch is not necessary since they are not affected by the dissection. The spermatic cord is taped. Contrary to what occurs in the Lichtenstein repair, no extensive dissection between the external oblique aponeurosis and internal oblique muscle is undertaken. The type of hernia is determined; spinal or local anesthesia can make it easier for the patient to strain and to cough.

In indirect hernias the cremaster is cut at its insertion around the deep inguinal orifice, to facilitate identification of the epigastric vessels at the medial margin, but it is not resected and it may be reinserted with a few stitches at the end of the procedure. The sac is dissected and reduced into the preperitoneal space. Blunt preperitoneal dissection is carried out through the internal orifice. It is initiated with a blunt curved clamp (e.g., Kelly clamp), just under the epigastric vessels, at the medial margin of the internal ring. Then a gauze is introduced through the deep orifice and dissection is extended with the index finger using this "dissection gauze". Dissection starts first medially, in the space of Retzius, up to the pubic bone. Then lateral dissection is carried out in the space of Bogros, up to the iliac spine or close to it. This lateral dissection may be a little bit more difficult, due to the tougher adherence between the peritoneum and abdominal wall, but it is achieved by proceeding gently with the finger and the moist dissection gauze.

The extent of dissection must be sufficient to accommodate the patch, but more extensive dissection is neither necessary nor useful. In practice, the length of the index finger in the direction of the pubis and in the direction of iliac spine, as well as the same in width, is adequate.

At the end of the dissection, the gauze is removed before proceeding to placement of the patch. The size of the patch (medium or large) is chosen according to anatomy.

The medial half of the patch (widest side) is introduced first in the direction of the pubic bone. To do so, one angled retractor lifts the epigastric vessels, another one (blade retractor) reclines the peritoneum medially, so that the Cooper's ligament becomes visible. The widest end of the patch, grasped with the Kelly clamp, is introduced in the direction of the pubis. Then, the clamp and retractors are removed.

To introduce the lateral part of the patch, two retractors lift the lateral edge of the internal orifice and, using a clamp in one hand and a toothless forceps in the other, the surgeon manages to gently introduce the lateral half of the patch in the lateral compartment of the preperitoneal space. Then, the retractors are removed and deployment of the patch is achieved with the finger by pushing on the memory-ring. The counter-pressure exerted by the patient straining can facilitate deployment. Asking the patient to strain helps check that the prosthetic patch has securely fixed the hernia bulge. In cases where a small protrusion still occurs this is easily corrected by readjusting the patch. For this reason, local or spinal anesthesia are good choices. Thanks to the abdominal pressure, the memory-ring and the limited dissection, no fixation of the patch is required. The external oblique aponeurosis, Scarpa's fascia and the skin are sutured.

In direct hernias a circular incision of the transversalis fascia is performed at the base of the sac and the sac is reduced. Then, preperitoneal dissection and placement of the patch are carried out through the fascia orifice. It should be emphasized that checking for a small unapparent indirect sac is mandatory, and that the lateral dissection is extended as far as for an indirect hernia, to parietalize the cord and correctly cover the lateral compartment. The procedure is very easy in the case of large mixed hernias in which both components are evident.

9.2.2 Tips and Tricks

The avascular preperitoneal plane of dissection is located between the deep aspect of the transversalis fascia and the preperitoneal fat, which is attached to the peritoneum. As small blood vessels are contained in the fat, they are not damaged when dissection is carried out in contact with the fascia. Therefore, for a bloodless dissection to be carried out, the finger pad or the blunt tip of the Kelly clamp must constantly face upwards and keep in contact with the fascia. This plane of dissection can be aided by infiltration of local anesthetic. As for major vessels, they are easily palpated and protected by the vascular sheath.

The "dissection gauze" is not intended to create the pocket by its volume, but it is used for blunt dissection, moved with the fingertip, like a gauze nut.

When switching from the dissection of medial to that of lateral compartment, changing hands can facilitate the gesture.

The gauze must be removed before introducing the patch, thus it may be useful to set two practical rules: 1) never use more than one gauze, 2) the nurse only gives the patch to the surgeon *after* the surgeon has given back the "dissection gauze".

When grasping the patch with a toothless clamp to introduce it medially, it is important that: 1) the clamp does not hold the memory-ring, 2) the clamp is positioned under the patch, so that the patch is bent over the clamp and its curvature fits with the convex shape of the peritoneal sac and the concave shape of the deep aspect of the abdominal wall. Doing so facilitates patch deployment.

When introducing the patch medially, do not follow the natural tendency to push it too far, because in this case covering of the lateral compartment will not be sufficient. Only the medial half of the patch – no more – is introduced medially.

When introducing the lateral end of the patch laterally, do not follow the natural tendency to push towards the umbilicus. The correct direction is towards the iliac spine.

Correct deployment of the lateral part of the patch is essential, because in the case it is not totally flat and the tip kinks up into the muscular wall, it may induce discomfort. If this occurs, a very simple solution can relieve such symptoms. A short skin incision (1-2 cm) located over the kink is performed in local anesthesia. A small opening of the funnel containing the memory-ring is performed with the scalpel or scissors and the plastic ring is easily pulled out.

The counter-pressure exerted by straining facilitates patch deployment. Therefore, spinal or local anesthesia is very useful. It is suggested to start these repairs under spinal or epidural anesthesia in the first instance.

9.2.3   Results

The TIPP repair fits well with day case surgery. In the initial series it was performed with an overnight stay in half of the cases, principally because of national regulation. However, in a recent French series the percentage of day surgery evolved with national rules and increased from 48% in 2010 to 72% in 2012 [7], and in the TULIP trial the majority of repairs were performed as day cases [8].

Postoperative pain is indeed tolerable. Pain assessed by visual analog scale was rated at 1.67/10 and 2.7/10 in two series [3, 5] and the percentage of patients who did not take analgesics was 6% and 15% [3, 9]. The time off work was around two weeks. Intraoperative events reported in one series [7] occurred in 4%. They included peritoneal tears and injury of epigastric vessels and were easily managed by peritoneum suture or vessel ligature. The percentage of postoperative complications was around 5-7%. All were benign superficial complications. There were 0.4 to 4% hematomas, but cases of severe bleeding have not been reported [4, 5, 7].

At a mean follow-up of two years, the recurrence rate was 0.4 to 1.5% [4, 5, 7]. In one study, three recurrences (2%) were diagnosed by systematic ultrasound, but they were not perceptible at physical examination [9], which makes their true significance debatable. No serious complications and no cases of testicular atrophy have been reported. The percentage of chronic pain ranged from 2.5% to 4.8% in two series [5, 9]. It was 7% in the initial evaluation but since the inventing surgeon wanted to be as objective as possible, this included one case of preoperative pain that remained unchanged after operation and three cases of pain that could clearly be related to causes other than surgery [4]. In the largest series looking at quality of life assessment, pain was globally rated as mild; only

0.8% of the patients rated their pain as severe, but they also declared they did not take any analgesics and that they experienced no impairment in professional and leisure activity, which suggests a possible misunderstanding of the rating scale used [7]. There was no case of debilitating pain and none of the patients took regular analgesics, with 97% considering their overall result as good or excellent.

The TULIP trial was a randomized double blind clinical trial comparing TIPP to Lichtenstein, using an accurate methodology, focused on reducing the risk of errors in the dimensions of bias, random error and the chosen outcome measures [8]. The operation time was shorter with the TIPP (34 minutes vs. 40 minutes). Postoperative complications were significantly fewer in the TIPP group (6.4% vs. 20.3%). Serious complications, especially bleeding, were not observed. Postoperative pain was not different in the two groups, probably because in both repairs the wound was infiltrated with local anesthetic. The mean time to resume activities of daily life, including work and sport, was significantly shorter for patients in the TIPP group (9.9 days vs. 16.4 days). The recurrence rate was not significantly different, though it was higher in the Lichtenstein group (2.6% vs. 1.4%). There were significantly fewer patients experiencing continuous chronic pain as well as activity-related pain in the TIPP group (3.6% and 8.5% respectively) than in the Lichtenstein group (12.9% and 38.5% respectively). The percentage of persisting numbness was higher with the Lichtenstein (49.7%) than with the TIPP repair (10.5%).

Evaluation of health status using the SF36 questionnaire showed that the dimensions of physical pain and physical functioning were better for patients operated on by TIPP than by Lichtenstein [10]. The economic evaluation concluded that from a hospital perspective there were no differences between the two methods, but from a societal perspective a significant difference in favor of the TIPP was found, with savings of 1,472 Euro, essentially because the time off work was shorter in the TIPP group [11].

9.2.4   Advantages of the TIPP

Preperitoneal location of the patch minimizes the risk of injury to the sensitive nerves running in the inguinal canal, when nerve injury is an essential factor of chronic pain. In the Lichtenstein procedure, the wide dissection of the inguinal canal necessary to deploy the patch, and the fixation required to resist intraabdominal pressure, can result in nerve damage. The crucial role of nerve damage may be underlined by the great number of publications aimed at dealing with nerve management, such as nerve identification, neurolysis, nerve resection, use of glue or self-adhesive patch.

Unfortunately, identification of all three nerves – especially the genital branch – is not always possible and neurolysis is even a risk factor of chronic pain [12]. Nerve entrapment by sutures may be avoided by using glue, but the results of meta-analyses are controversial, the efficacy of glue to minimize chronic pain is not really established and self-adhesive patches do not do any better [12]. All of this is understandable, since glue can prevent nerve entrapment by sutures, but not the chronic inflammatory reaction induced by the patch, which can involve and damage the nerves, as demonstrated by an experimental study on rabbits [13]. An inguinal approach is a risk factor for chronic pain *per se* [12], but this was established by studies that did not include the TIPP. The case may very well be different with the TIPP, since dissection of the inguinal canal is limited, the patch does not come into contact with the nerves and no fixation is required. The superiority of the TIPP has been clearly demonstrated by the TULIP trial with a low risk of bias [8, 10].

The benefits of the preperitoneal patch have been demonstrated by two high-quality randomized trials, which showed that the total extraperitoneal approach (TEP) provided better results than the Lichtenstein and concluded that TEP could be recommended as the optimal technique in experienced hands [14–16]. Reference to the surgeon's skill is important, because of the limitations of laparoscopic techniques. Laparoscopy does indeed require general anesthesia with deep relaxation, it is more demanding than open techniques, the learning curve is longer and it can induce more complications. TIPP is easier: in the TULIP trial, surgery was performed by senior surgeons assisted by residents as well as by residents assisted by senior surgeons, and the mean operation time was 34 minutes.

TIPP does not require general anesthesia with curare. It can be performed with a laryngeal mask without curare [7], or with spinal anesthesia. It can also be carried out in local anesthesia with sedation, provided correct infiltration of the preperitoneal space is performed using a sufficient volume of 0.5% lidocaine, rather than a smaller volume or long-action anesthetics [17]. Intraoperative events are easily managed and the operating duration is less variable than with laparoscopy, which facilitates the planning of operative room and day surgery unit. For these reasons, Gillion and Chollet who had a large experience with the TEP, switched to the TIPP as their preferred method of repair [7].

Another advantage of the TIPP is that switching to another technique, when dissection of the preperitoneal space is difficult due to a history of preperitoneal surgery, can easily be carried out through the same incision. In one series, this was the case in a patient who had a sacral trauma with extensive bleeding some months earlier [5]. In another series, preperitoneal dissection was possible in 8 of 17 cases with a history of urologic or vascular surgery, but it was not possible in 9 cases, which were solved by a Lichtenstein or a plug [17]. TIPP is the only technique of preperitoneal repair that allows conversion without having to perform an additional incision.

Contrary to laparoscopy that involves a large dissection and a wide overlapping of the patch on the iliac vessels, TIPP requires less extensive dissection. Only the preperitoneal pocket necessary to accommodate the patch is created and the contact between the patch and the iliac vessels is indeed minimal.

9.3 The TREPP (Transrectus Sheath Extraperitoneal Procedure) Technique

The TREPP technique was developed by Akkersdijk, based on five principles [18]:
- use a simple, easy-to-learn, open technique
- stay away from the nerves in the inguinal canal during dissection
- mesh positioning in the preperitoneal space, away from nerves
- no need for mesh fixation
- neither dissection nor reconstruction of the inguinal canal.

A description of the technique and preliminary results has been published [18, 19]. The operation is performed under spinal or general anesthesia. The incision is carried out one finger above the line between the pubic tubercle and iliac spine, following Langer's lines. It starts about 1 cm lateral to the midline with a total length of about 6 cm. The anterior rectus sheath is divided parallel to the incision and the rectus muscle is retracted medially. At this level the transversalis fascia is a thin conjunctive layer that is easily divided. The inferior epigastric vessels are also retracted medially.

Preperitoneal dissection is started medially in the space of Retzius and then extended laterally in the space of Bogros. A preperitoneal pocket is created, limited by the abdominal wall ventrally, the psoas muscle dorsolaterally and the iliac vessels medially. The peritoneum and the indirect sac are separated from the cord elements. They are reclined dorsally with a retractor, whereas the cord elements stay applied on the abdominal wall.

In case of a direct hernia, reduction of the sac is easily achieved by dissection of the space of Retzius, but lateral dissection and cord parietalization must be achieved to allow correct deployment of the patch.

The Polysoft patch is introduced and easily deployed, applied onto the abdominal wall, patching all three areas of potential weakness. As a consequence of the memory-ring and the effect of abdominal pressure, no fixation is necessary. Only the anterior rectus sheath and skin require suturing.

The preliminary results on 1000 cases are promising [19]. Only 19 benign postoperative complications occurred; there were no cases of severe complications and particularly no case of serious bleeding.

There were 11 recurrences (1.2%) and 49 cases of chronic pain, but only four patients took analgesics and most patients with chronic pain already suffered from pain prior to operation. Ninety-eight percent of patients declared they were satisfied with their operation.

TREPP seems indeed to be a promising technique, due to the absence of any sort of damage to the inguinal nerves, because they are endangered neither by the dissection nor by the contact with the patch. Nevertheless, the results of the randomized trial, currently in process (ISRCTN18591339), are awaited.

9.4 The ONSTEP (Open New Simplified Totally Extraperitoneal) Technique

ONSTEP was developed by Lourenço and da Costa [20]. In this technique the medial half of the Polysoft patch is introduced into the preperitoneal space through an opening in the transversalis fascia and the lateral half is placed between the external oblique aponeurosis and the internal oblique muscle. The patch is split to accommodate the spermatic cord and the arms of the split are simply approximated by three stitches. The main advantage of ONSTEP is that the technique may be easier to perform than the TIPP, because it avoids dissection of the lateral compartment of the preperitoneal space. This technique is described by Rosenberg and Andresen in another chapter of this book.

9.5 Future Developments

In April 2015 a new patch called ONFLEX, equipped with an absorbable memory-ring was launched. In accordance with the original concept, only the flat large-pore mesh will remain in place after the memory-ring is absorbed. Consequently, it may be that tolerance will be improved and kinking of the lateral extremity of the patch will no longer be a problem, but at the expense of the spring effect.

References

1. Pélissier EP, Blum D, Marre P et al (2001) Inguinal hernia: a patch covering only the myopectineal orifice is effective. Hernia 5:84–87
2. Pélissier EP (2006) Inguinal hernia: preperitoneal placement of a memory-ring patch by anterior approach. Preliminary experience. Hernia 10:248–252
3. Pélissier EP, Monek O, Blum D et al (2007) The Polysoft patch: prospective evaluation of feasibility, postoperative pain and recovery. Hernia 11:229–234
4. Pélissier EP, Blum D, Ngo P et al (2008) Transinguinal preperitoneal repair with the Polysoft patch: prospective evaluation of recurrence and chronic pain. Hernia 12:51–56
5. Berrevoet F, Sommeling C, De Gendt S et al (2009) The preperitoneal memory-ring patch for inguinal hernia: a prospective multicentric feasibility study. Hernia 13:243–249
6. Pélissier EP (2009) Preperitoneal memory-ring patch for inguinal hernia. Re: Preperitoneal memory-ring patch for inguinal hernia: a prospective multicentric feasibility study, Berrevoet et al (2009). Hernia 13:451–452
7. Gillion JF, Chollet JM (2013) Chronic pain and quality of life (QoL) after transinguinal preperitoneal (TIPP) inguinal hernia repair using a totally extraperitoneal, parietalized, Polysoft memory ring patch: a series of 622 hernia repairs in 525 patients. Hernia 17:683–692
8. Koning GG, Keus F, Koeslag L et al (2012) Randomized clinical trial of chronic pain after the transinguinal preperitoneal technique compared with Lichtenstein's method for inguinal hernia repair. Br J Surg 99:1365–1373
9. Maillart JF, Vantournhoudt P, Piret-Gerard G et al (2011) Transinguinal preperitoneal groin hernia repair using a preperitoneal mesh preformed with a permanent memory ring: a good alternative to Lichtenstein's technique. Hernia 15:289–295

10. Koning GG, de Vries J, Borm GF et al (2013) Health status one year after Transinguinal preperitoneal inguinal hernia repair and Lichtenstein's method: an analysis alongside a randomized clinical study. Hernia 17:299–306

11. Koning GG, Adang EM, Stalmeier PF et al (2013) TIPP and Lichtenstein modalities for inguinal hernia repair: a cost minimisation analysis alongside a randomised trial. Eur J Health Econ 14:1027–1034

12. Bjurstrom MF, Nicol AL, Amid PK et al (2014) Pain control following inguinal herniorrhaphy: current perspectives. J Pain Res 7:277–290

13. Demirer S, Kepenekci I, Evirgen O et al (2006) The effect of polypropylene mesh on ilioinguinal nerve in open mesh repair of groin hernia. J Surg Res 131:175–181

14. Langeveld HR, van't Riet M, Weidema WF et al (2010) Total extraperitoneal inguinal hernia repair compared with Lichtenstein (the LEVEL-Trial): a randomized controlled trial. Ann Surg 251:819–824

15. Eker HH, Langeveld HR, Klitsie PJ et al (2012) Randomized clinical trial of total extraperitoneal inguinal hernioplasty vs Lichtenstein repair: a long-term follow-up study. Arch Surg 147:256–260

16. Eklund A, Montgomery A, Bergkvist L et al (2010) Chronic pain 5 years after randomized comparison of laparoscopic and Lichtenstein inguinal hernia repair. Br J Surg 97:600–608

17. Pélissier EP, Ngo P, Gayet B (2011) Transinguinal preperitoneal patch (TIPP) under local anesthesia with sedation. Am Surg 77:1681–1684

18. Koning GG, Andeweg CS, Keus F et al (2012) The transrectus sheath preperitoneal mesh repair for inguinal hernia: technique, rationale, and results of the first 50 cases. Hernia 16:295–259

19. Lange JF, Lange MM, Voropai DA et al (2014) Trans rectus sheath extra-peritoneal procedure (TREPP) for inguinal hernia: the first 1,000 patients. World J Surg 38:1922–1928

20. Lourenço A, da Costa RS (2013) The ONSTEP inguinal hernia repair technique: initial clinical experience of 693 patients, in two institutions. Hernia 17:357–364

A video demonstrating TIPP in local anesthesia is available on MEDtube:

Pélissier E, Ngo P (2015) Inguinal Hernia Repair by Transinguinal Preperitoneal Patch in Local Anesthesia https://medtube.net/general-surgery/medical-videos/16803-inguinal-hernia-repair-by-transinguinal-preperitoneal-patch-in-local-anesthesia

Minimal Open Preperitoneal (MOPP) Technique

10

Marc Soler

10.1 Introduction

The use of a large preperitoneal prosthesis to treat groin hernias was proposed more than 50 years ago by Nyhus [1]. Wantz [2] with the same concept presented a transrectal procedure, which would allow, according to the author's wishes, the treatment of complex hernias (e.g., recurrent hernias) under local anesthesia in an ambulatory setting, but it was not possible to do it in practice.

The Ugahary technique [3, 4] achieved this ambition by combining the concept of visceral sac reinforcement by means of a large Stoppa prosthesis [5] with Ugahary's concept of minimally invasive surgery (small grid iron incision). However, for many authors, the realization was difficult to reproduce and difficult to teach.

The new Pélissier [6] prosthesis with a rigid peripheral ring has made the transinguinal preperitoneal (TIPP) technique possible.

Our minimal open preperitoneal (MOPP) technique is a TIPP technique that uses the Ugahary principle of preperitoneal space dissection with specific retractors (Fig. 10.1), through a 3-4 cm incision (Fig. 10.2). The main principle of MOPP is to unroll a large prosthesis far beyond the limits of the Fruchaud's myopectineal orifice. The prosthesis is applied against the abdominal wall by the underlying pressure. The incision is next to the deep inguinal ring (Fig. 10.2). The anesthesia can be local or with an ilioinguinal or transversus abdominis plane (TAP) block. In our practice we use general anesthesia with a laryngeal mask without intubation and without curarization, associated with local anesthesia. The instrumentation (Fig. 10.1) is simple but specifically dedicated. Rapid return to normal activities is an advantage of the technique, contributing to its low cost. When the general conditions allow, the procedure is performed as a day case

M. Soler (✉)
Centre de Chirurgie Pariétale
Cagnes sur Mer, France
e-mail: soler.marc2@wanadoo.fr

G. Campanelli (Ed), *Inguinal Hernia Surgery,*
Updates in Surgery
DOI: 10.1007/978-88-470-3947-6_10, © Springer-Verlag Italia 2017

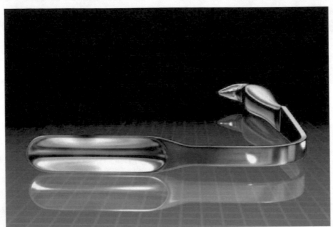

Fig. 10.1 Specific retractor

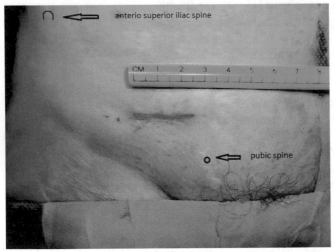

Fig. 10.2 MOPP incision

(in more than 90% in our practice). Preoperative preparation and precautions are standard and show no specificity.

10.2 Prosthesis and Instrumentation

The prosthesis is selected according to the need to be unrolled in the preperitoneal space, through a small incision. A wide polypropylene mesh prosthesis has been specifically devised for this technique; it has a peripheral hem with a reinforcement (Fig. 10.3) to facilitate proper deployment of the prosthesis. The prosthesis is

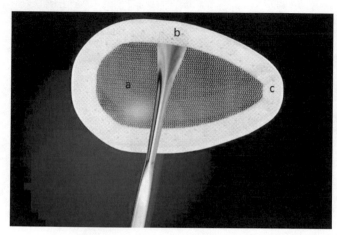

Fig. 10.3 The MOPP prosthesis. **a** Large pore size polypropylene mesh. **b** Non-knitted non-woven peripheral reinforcement. **c** Peripheral hem

available in two sizes, 16.5 cm/12 cm and 13.5 cm/9 cm. The quality of the prosthesis allows for the minimally invasive technique. This technique requires some very long and narrow retractors (Fig. 10.1) allowing a wide and deep dissection. A long dressing forceps with an atraumatic end is used to introduce the prosthesis behind the pubic bone, in contact with the bladder, without any risk of causing injury to it.

10.3 Surgical Technique

10.3.1 The Minimal Open Route Between the Skin and the Deep Inguinal Ring

The skin incision (Fig. 10.2) is deliberately small. With experience it can be between 25 and 40 mm. It lies immediately in front of the deep inguinal ring. Several landmarks can be drawn on the patient's skin. The easiest approach is to simply connect the superior anterior iliac spine to the pubic tubercle and draw the incision transversely to the union of the internal and middle third.

After incision of the skin and subcutaneous layers, the fascia of the external oblique muscle is incised in line with its fibers. The ilioinguinal nerve is generally identified and preserved.

The spermatic cord is dissected (Fig. 10.4), separating the funicular pedicle (the blue line) which is left behind. Time to time it is necessary to separate an old and fibrous medial sac from the spermatic cord. The cord is also separating from the ilio inguinal nerve. I never cut the cremaster fibers: they are retracted medially. At this step, a lateral hernia sac is sought: locating a large and old sac is easy, but sometimes you find a small sac in the most proximal part of the cord.

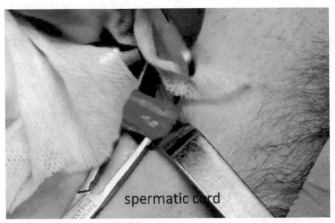

Fig. 10.4 Externalization of the spermatic cord

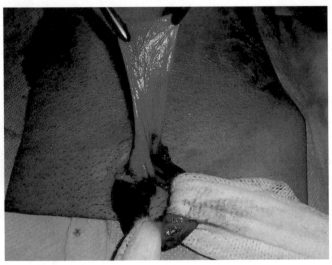

Fig. 10.5 Individualization of the lateral hernia sac

The lateral sac is separated from the cord (Fig. 10.5). Similarly, a lipoma of the cord will also be dissected and resected, as its persistence may be responsible for postoperative pain, sometimes feeling like a pseudo recurrence. Parietalization of the sac is initiated, pushing it through the deep inguinal orifice.

10.3.2 Cleavage of the Preperitoneal Space

Penetration into the peritoneal space starts through the deep inguinal ring, laterally to the epigastric vessels, previously identified (Fig. 10.6). Cleavage of the preperitoneal space is initiated (Fig. 10.7), back to the transversalis fascia

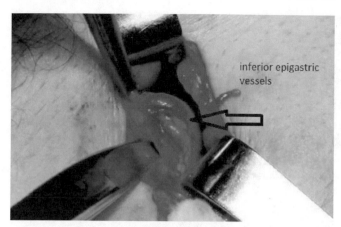

Fig. 10.6 Inferior epigastric vessels identified

inferior epigastric
vessels

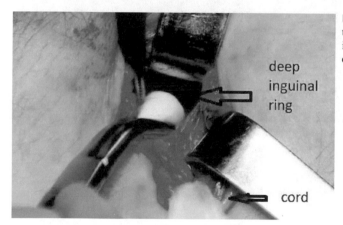

Fig. 10.7 Cleavage of
the preperitoneal space
is initiated through the
deep inguinal ring

deep
inguinal
ring

cord

– which is very fine at this location – pushing it medially and progressing back
to the inferior epigastric vessels; the vessels are pressed against the anterior
abdominal wall, where they will be well protected throughout the procedure with
a retractor. Using the dedicated retractors (Fig.10.8), the dissection extends into
the avascular plane medially and laterally along the inferior epigastric vessels in
the direction of the iliac vessels, quickly and easily, cleaving the spaces of Retzius
and Bogros. Cooper's ligament is easily spotted, the bladder pushed back, and the
retropubic space is cleared (Fig. 10.9). Dissection of the space for accommodating
the prosthesis continues inwards and upwards with retractors of increasing size.
Facing the upper edge of the incision, the peritoneum may be more adherent to the
superficial plane and must be gradually separated with scissors; it is imperative
to widely open the plane at this level. The top and posterior dissection is easier to
widely explore the psoas muscle.

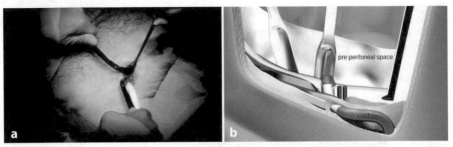

Fig. 10.8 a Dissection of the preperitoneal space with the specific retractors. **b** Dissection of the preperitoneal space with the specific retractors, synthetic image

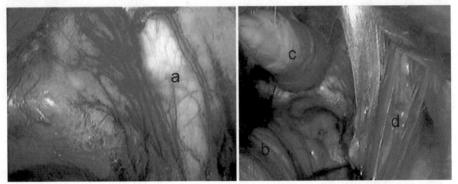

Fig. 10.9 Dissected preperitoneal space. **a** Cooper's ligament. **b** Bladder. **c** Visceral sac. **d** Spermatic cord with a large lateral sac

10.3.3 Parietalization of the Spermatic Cord

The elements of the spermatic cord should be separated from the peritoneum, about 10 cm relative to the deep inguinal ring, so as to achieve parietalization of the cord (Fig. 10.10). During the dissection, the spermatic sheet described by R. Stoppa [7], uniting the vas deferens medially and the spermatic vessels laterally, must be carefully respected, if possible. After parietalization, this spermatic fascia can be interposed between the prosthesis and the external iliac vessels. After dissection of the cord, the "parietalization triangle", of which the summit is the spermatic cord, the medial edge the vas deferens, and the lateral edge the spermatic vessels, is well exposed (Fig. 10.11).

10.3.4 Placing the Prosthesis

We use a mesh having a peripheral reinforcement with a non-rigid hem (Fig. 10.3). The dissected preperitoneal space is held open by three retractors (Fig. 10.12). One of the retractors raises the anterior abdominal wall thereby protecting

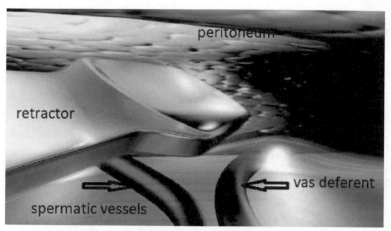

Fig. 10.10 Parietalization of the spermatic cord with the specific retractors, synthetic image

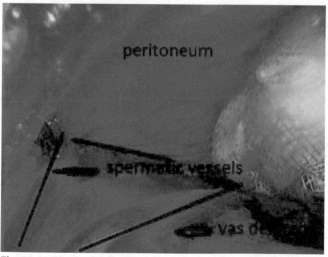

Fig. 10.11 The "parietalization triangle"

the epigastric vessels, the other two long and narrow retractors push back the visceral sac and the bladder.

To prepare for the introduction of the prosthesis, we use an atraumatic clamp (dressing forceps) that gauges the distance between the retropubic region released and the incision. The prosthesis is grasped with this atraumatic forceps at the middle part of its lower and median edge, and introduced through the incision parallel to the inguinal ligament, up retropubic region, taking into account the previously obtained measurement (Fig. 10.12).

The same forceps is used to grasps the upper and lateral part of the prosthesis and introduce it in the upper and lateral portion of the preperitoneal dissection

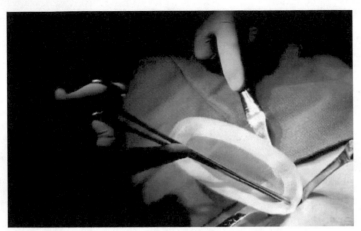

Fig. 10.12 Introduction of the mesh with the dressing forceps

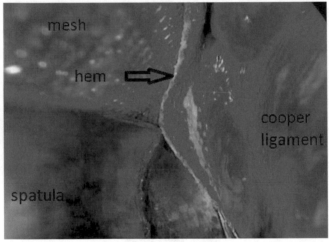

Fig. 10.13 Checking and improvement of the correct position of the prosthesis using a spatula

area. The lower end of the prosthesis is placed behind the pubis. The upper end is placed in front of the psoas muscle. The prosthesis is thus partially deployed in the dissection space. Expansion of the prosthesis is completed by using retractors, finger, and forceps. The correct position of the prosthesis can be controlled and improved by using a spatula instrument, which can move along the hem of the prosthesis and possibly remove any folds, thus optimizing good spreading out of its periphery (Fig. 10.13).

The prosthesis is never fixed. When positioning of the prosthesis is satisfactory, the spermatic cord is reintroduced under the external oblique muscle fascia.

Once the prosthesis is in place, the operator sees the deep inguinal ring spontaneously close partially, "like a sphincter". It is not necessary to suture the musculofascial plane. During closure of the external oblique aponeurosis, the ilioinguinal nerve is carefully avoided. The subcutaneous plane is closed with two reversing stitches, and adhesive strips are applied to the skin.

Showering is permitted the following day. An adhesive bandage protects the adhesive strips; this is changed every day, and requires no special care until final removal of the strips on day 10.

10.4   Indications

All primary, inguinal or femoral hernias can be treated by this technique, in particular large scrotal inguinal hernias (Fig.10.14) or femoral hernias (Fig. 10.15).

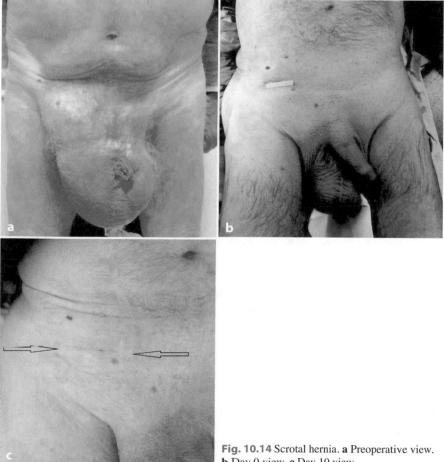

Fig. 10.14 Scrotal hernia. a Preoperative view. b Day 0 view. c Day 10 view

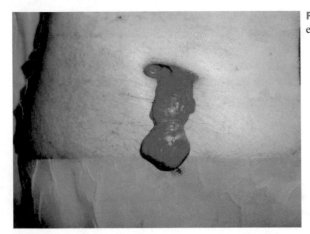

Fig. 10.15 Femoral hernia, externalization of the hernia sac

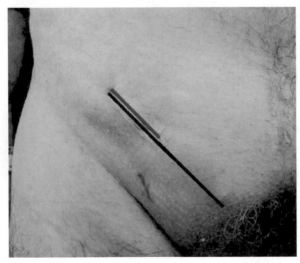

Fig. 10.16 Recurrent hernia after Lichtenstein. *Black line*, the initial Lichtenstein incision. *Red line*, the adapted MOPP incision to treat the recurrence

In the presence of bilateral hernia, both sides are operated on in the same operating session, and the two prostheses are superimposed on the midline. Recurrent hernias without material previously established in the preperitoneal space are a very good indication. Recurrent hernias after Lichtenstein are also an excellent indication (Fig. 10.16), with the possibility of setting up a new prosthesis, the preperitoneal space is often free of adhesion. If the previous prosthesis is retained, sometimes a plug must be resected.

10.5 Special Cases

10.5.1 Female Hernias

The round ligament is always distally dissected and sectioned, it is largely repressed with a possible external oblique sac.

10.5.2 Femoral Hernia

This is an excellent indication for the technique, it is easy to expand the femoral ring with the finger and repress back fringes incarcerated fat. In its normal position, the prosthesis covers widely the femoral hole and the obturator foramen.

10.5.3 Scrotal Hernia

It is easy to dissect step by step a bulky inguinal scrotal sac, the distal part of the sac may be dropped in the scrotum.

10.5.4 Strangulated Hernia

It is also possible to treat a strangulated hernia. An intestinal loop can be resected if necessary, through an enlarged transverse incision. Then it is possible to complete the operation by the same way with or without using prosthetic material.

10.6 Contraindications

Previous radical prostatectomy, pelvic irradiation, or realization of a vascular bypass with dissection of the preperitoneal space can be a contraindication of the MOPP technique, as are recurrent hernias with prosthesis implanted in the preperitoneal space. However, with experience, even in these situations it is often possible to start with the MOPP technique and, in the case of failure of the preperitoneal dissection, continue with the Lichtenstein technique with the same incision. It is not a conversion.

10.7   Personal Data

A total of 778 hernias were operated on between September 2011 and June 2015. All cases were treated in an ambulatory setting. Our results have been good, with few complications and no cases of reoperation (Table 10.1). Satisfaction at 2 years is excellent. There have been no cases of recurrence during this period. Pain was rated on VAS (Visual Analog Scale), and the rate of severe postoperative pain is very low (Table 10.2). Only 97 patients reporting pain at 1 month were reviewed at 3 months (Table 10.2). For four patients, postoperative pain was worse than preoperative pain, but no medication or limitation of activity was required.

Table 10.1 Baseline demographic characteristics and outcome of 778 hernias operated between September 2011 to June 2015

Hernias operated	778	
Mean follow-up	711 days	
Technique	MOPP 644 Ugahary 74 Lichtenstein 25	
About MOPP	Patients 534	Men 483 (90.45%), Women 51 (9.55%)
	Hernias 644	Unilateral 424 (79.40%), Bilateral 220 (20.60%)
	Type of hernia	Lateral 401 (62.26%) Medial 251 (38.97%) Femoral 28 (4.34%): Female 16, Men 12
	Prosthesis N=619	Large size (16.5/12 cm) ovoid polypropylen mesh 260 (42%) Medium size (13.5/9 cm) ovoid polypropylen mesh, 359 (58%)
	Length of stay	Day case 598 (92.8%) One night stay 30 (4.64%) More than one night 13 (2.01%)
	Complications	Bladder retention 2 Phlebitis 1 Superficial infection 2 Deep infection 0 Reoperation 0
	At two years N=220	No discomfort 214(97.27%) Discomfort 5(2.27%) Moderate pain 1(0.45%) Satisfaction: Excellent 212, Medium 1 No recurrence

Table 10.2 Postoperative pain and chronic pain at days 8, 30, and 90, based on VAS scores (visual analog scale)

	Day 8	Day 30	Day 90
N	624	553	97
VAS 0	337 (54%)	452 (81.73%)	77 (79.38%)
VAS 1-3	225 (36.05%)	77 (13.92%)	9 (927%)
VAS 4-6	57 (9.13%)	19 (3.43%)	10 (10.30%)
VAS 7-8	8 (1.28%)	5 (0.90%)	1 (1%)

10.8   Conclusions

The MOPP technique is a minimal open preperitoneal technique using a large wide mesh. Nearly all kinds of groin hernias, and all adult patients, can be treated. A frail elderly patient with a large hernia is a good indication as anesthesia can be adapted.

The patients are preferably treated in an ambulatory setting according to the usual criteria and precautions. There are no particular restrictions regarding the allowed postoperative activities. Our data show a low rate of chronic pain and no cases of recurrence.

References

1. Nyhus LM, Condon RE, Harkins HN (1960) Clinical experience with preperitoneal hernia repair for all kinds of hernia of the groin. Am J Surg 100:234–244
2. Wantz GE, Fischer E (2001) Unilateral giant prosthetic reinforcement of visceral sac: Preperitoneal hernioplasties with Dacron. In: Bendavid R (ed) Abdominal wall hernias. Principles and management. Springer, New York, pp 396–400
3. Ugahary F, Simmermacher RKF (1998) Groin hernia repair via a grid-iron incision year alternative technique for preperitoneal mesh incision. Hernia 2:123–125
4. Soler M, Ugahary F (2004) Cure des hernies de l'aine par grande prothèse prépéritonéale par voie inguinale supérieure et latérale (technique de Ugahary). E-mémoires de l'Académie Nationale de Chirurgie 3:28–33
5. Stoppa R, Petit J, Abourachid H et al (1973) Procédé original de plastie des hernies de l'aine: l'interposition sans fixation d'une prothèse en tulle de Dacron par voie médiane sous-péritonéal. Chirurgie 99:119–123
6. Pélissier EP (2006) Inguinal hernia: preperitoneal placement of a memory-patch ring by anterior approach. Preliminary experience. Hernia 10:248–252
7. Stoppa R, Diarra B, Mertl P (1997) The retroparietal spermatic sheath. An anatomical structure of surgical interest. Hernia 1:55–59

Transabdominal Preperitoneal Patch (TAPP) 11

Jan F. Kukleta

One has to change something
sometimes in order to improve.

11.1 Introduction

The success of laparoscopic cholecystectomy in the late 80s led to an extension of the minimally invasive technique to one of the most frequent elective surgical procedures – groin hernia repair. After several ineffective and wrong laparoscopic concepts of obstructing the hernia orifice had obviously failed, the giant preperitoneal reinforcement of the visceral sac (GPVRS), an anterior open technique proposed and practiced by René Stoppa [1], attracted the interest of innovative laparo-endoscopic surgeons. Moving away from closing the hernia defects by sutured repair and towards the so-called tension-free repair, Stoppa covered the myopectineal orifice of Fruchaud [2] using a large polyester mesh interposed between the two layers of peritoneum - the visceral sac (peritoneum viscerale) and the endoabdominal fascia (peritoneum parietale). He reinforced the peritoneum with a mesh-scar-complex to make it inextensible in order to prevent further sac formation. Endoscopic surgeons, however, reinforce the muscular wall with the same mesh-scar complex supported by Pascal's hydrostatic principle (unique distribution of the intra-abdominal pressure) and this way bridge the hernia defects. By lowering the peak pressures the hernia creating force is used to support the mesh fixation and to prevent a recurrence.

Three endoscopic techniques using a posterior approach were developed in the early 90s: the transabdominal preperitoneal patch (TAPP), the totally extraperitoneal plasty (TEP) and the intraperitoneal onlay mesh (IPOM). The latter did not use the advantage of dissection of the preperitoneal space, retraction of hernia sacs or preperitoneal lipomas, but placed the non-absorbable prosthetic mesh upon the defect. The intraperitoneal mesh exposes viscera to potential morbidity. IPOM for inguinofemoral hernias is an inappropriate and ineffective therapy from today's perspective.

J.F. Kukleta (✉)
Visceral Surgery Unit, Hirslanden Klinik Im Park
Zurich, Switzerland
e-mail: jfkukleta@bluewin.ch

G. Campanelli (Ed), *Inguinal Hernia Surgery,*
Updates in Surgery
DOI: 10.1007/978-88-470-3947-6_11, © Springer-Verlag Italia 2017

The objective of minimal invasive preperitoneal groin hernia repair is the deployment of a large non-absorbable mesh in a widely dissected preperitoneal space covering and overlapping all potential inguinofemoral defects. Both TAPP and TEP reach the same final objective in different ways.

11.2   History of TAPP

The first report was published by Arregui [3] in 1992. As the TEP technique promoted by Dulucq, Ferzli and McKernan [4–6] became known at the same time and its performance was even more difficult than the TAPP repair, the reaction of the surgical community was disappointed and overwhelmed. Both TAPP and TEP are technically demanding techniques, TEP with an obviously longer and steeper learning curve.

Tension-free repairs brought many advantages (e.g., lower recurrence rates, less pain, fewer infections and earlier resumption of daily activities), but the prosthetic mesh became a must as a central pillar of the repair. This was initially one of the reasons for slow adoption, because of insufficient knowledge of mesh-host interaction; later on the meshes became the obvious part of a hernia repair irrespective of the approach. The lack of expertise in laparo-endoscopic repairs created new morbidities (e.g., vascular and intestinal lesions, bladder injury).

11.3   The Standardized TAPP [7]

11.3.1   Pneumoperitoneum

Establishing pneumoperitoneum enlarges the preexistent abdominal cavity and offers from the very start a spacious working environment. The exploration of the lower and upper abdomen allows for inspection of the initial pathology, of the contralateral groin and the remaining anterior aspect of intraabdominal content (Figs. 11.1–11.3).

11.3.2   Dissection

The preperitoneal space is entered through a planned incision of the visceral peritoneum way above the visible hernia defect not tailored to hernia type and size (Figs. 11.4 and 11.5). The complex preperitoneal anatomy is best described by Sakurai [8, 9]. Peeling of the visceral leaf from the parietal leaf (the latter protecting the underlying lower epigastric vessels in the form of an "endoabdominal" fascia) starts laterally in a fairly avascular plane supported by the "pneumodissection" of CO_2 gas under a pressure of 12 mmHg. We enter the space of Bogros (Fig. 11.6).

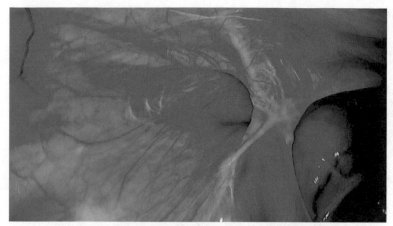

Fig. 11.1 Left indirect inguinal hernia

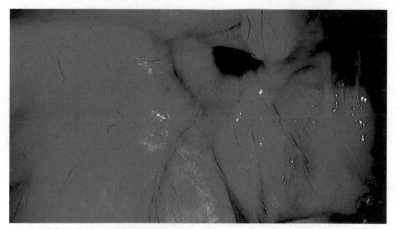

Fig. 11.2 Left direct inguinal hernia

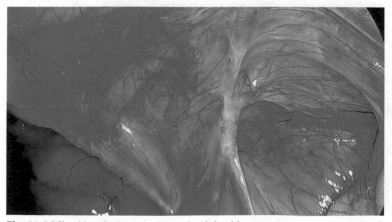

Fig. 11.3 Mixed hernia (pantaloon) on the right side

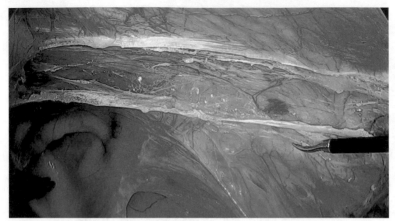

Fig. 11.4 Peritoneal incision above the defect on the right side

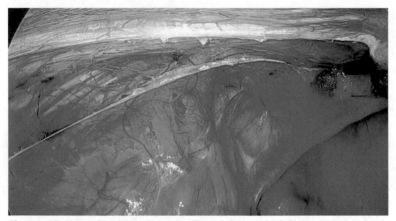

Fig. 11.5 Peritoneal incision above the direct defect on the left

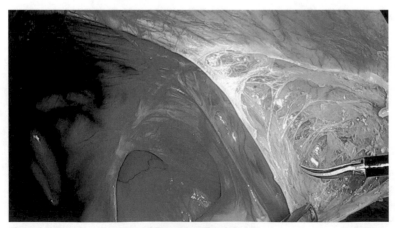

Fig. 11.6 Entering the space of Bogros on the right

Crossing the epigastric vessels in a medial direction, the endoabdominal fascia may continue to be a thin barrier which has to be entered to reach another spider-web-like compartment – the space of Retzius. These two anatomical spaces are not a continuation of each other, because they are not on the same level [9]. Further dissection deeper and medially finds Cooper's ligament and the superior pubic arch (Fig. 11.7) up to the landmark of the symphysis pubis. The dissection 1-2 cm beyond the midline is the medial margin of the so-called "landing zone". Caudally and laterally to the origin of the epigastric vessels and the inner inguinal ring, the figure of "A" is encountered (Figs. 11.8 and 11.9). The medial arm is the vas deferens complex and the lateral one the spermatic vessels. This region is often called the "triangle of doom" (because of the underlying external iliac vessels) (Fig. 11.10). Medial to the spermatic cord, a vascular anomaly of the arterial or venous

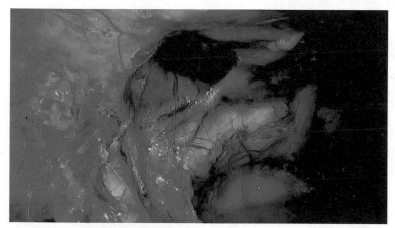

Fig. 11.7 Left direct hernia dissected

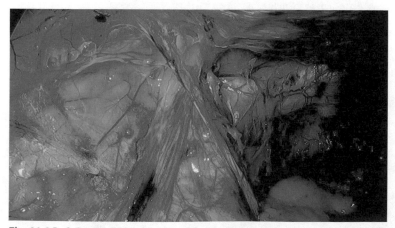

Fig. 11.8 Left figure of "A": triangle of doom

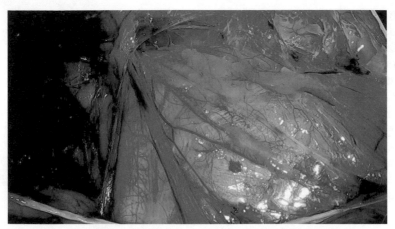

Fig. 11.9 Preserved spermatic fascia over triangle of pain on the right

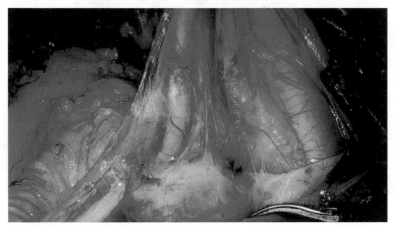

Fig. 11.10 Delicate dissection in triangle of doom on the right, vas deferens

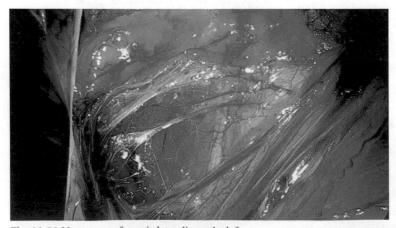

Fig. 11.11 N. cutaneus femoris lateralis on the left

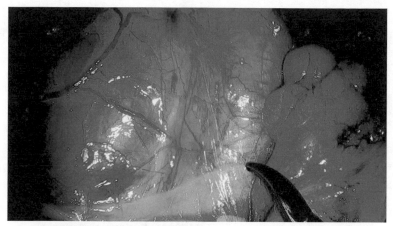

Fig. 11.12 Genitofemoral nerve on the left

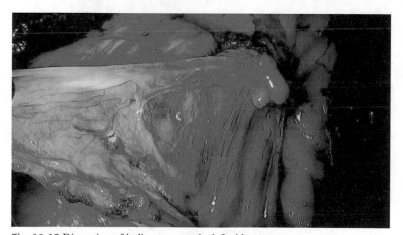

Fig. 11.13 Dissection of indirect sac on the left side

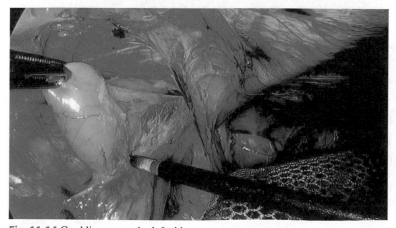

Fig. 11.14 Cord lipoma on the left side

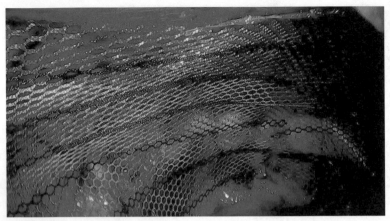

Fig. 11.15 Two separate meshes overlapping the symphysis pubis, left view

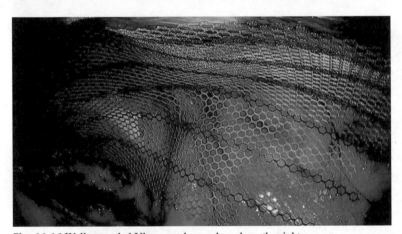

Fig. 11.16 Well-extended Ultrapro advanced mesh on the right

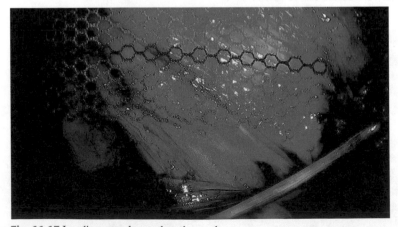

Fig. 11.17 Landing zone larger than the mesh

corona mortis (or both) anastomosis between the iliac and the obturator vessels can be found in about 20% of the population. The femoral canal is encountered between the iliopubic tract, Cooper's ligament and the external iliac vein. Lateral to the origin of the epigastric vessels the top of figure of "A" enters the inguinal canal. Laterally to the spermatic vessels a fat pad covers some nerves of the lumbar plexus (the genitofemoral nerve, the lateral cutaneous femoris and the femoral nerve) (Figs. 11.11 and 11.12). This area is called the triangle of pain. A very thin tissue layer covers both triangles and protects the fragile underlying structures in the form of the spermatic fascia. The dissection plane between the visceral and parietal peritoneal leaf facilitates the recognition and preservation of the spermatic fascia, which lowers the risk of postoperative nerve irritation or chronic pain. This gesture is easier to be accomplished in TAPP rather than in TEP, thanks to the preexisting working space and fearless dissection of the visceral leaf. In the case of dissectional insecurity, the TAPP technique allows the immediate view of the intraperitoneal structures behind the flap thereby avoiding possible sectional or thermal damage. After retraction of all hernia sacs and preperitoneal fat (Figs. 11.7 and 11.13) the presence of a cord lipoma has to be excluded. Substantial lipomas should be removed out of the inguinal canal because they are or may become symptomatic (Fig. 11.14). In large direct hernias, the remaining defect after retraction of the preperitoneal fat leaves a dead space behind. This predisposes to seroma formation and represents a risk factor for potential mesh dislocation. The attenuated transversalis fascia can be inverted and fixed with a suture or endo-loop in order to reduce this risk. The indirect sac should be retracted completely out the inguinal canal whenever possible. This sometimes difficult maneuver is safer after identification and dissection of the spermatic vessels.

11.3.3 Mesh Placement

Once the correct extent of the landing zone is achieved and hemostasis is secured an adequate mesh is inserted. According to the EHS [10] and the IEHS guidelines [7], today "adequate" means: a 15 × 10 cm or larger, macroporous flat mesh. The former criterion of weight per m² was substituted by the term "effective porosity", indicating the extent and quality of the tissue ingrowth. The mesh should be placed wrinkle- and fold-free (Figs. 11.15 and 11.16) respecting the well-defined anatomic landmarks. Especially the inferior mesh margin has to show a safety distance from the lowest lateral dissection area of the "landing zone" in order to prevent its lifting-up when closing the peritoneum (Fig. 11.17).

11.3.4 Fixation

The next step is still controversial. There is an evidence-based insight that not all preperitoneal hernia repairs require a mesh fixation. To fix the mesh to the

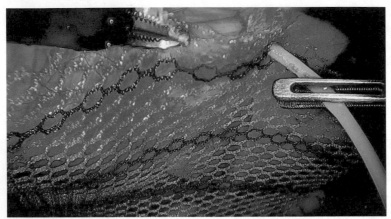

Fig. 11.18 Dropwise fixation with cyanoacrylate glue

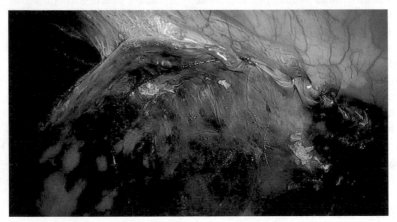

Fig. 11.19 Running suture to approximate the peritoneal flaps

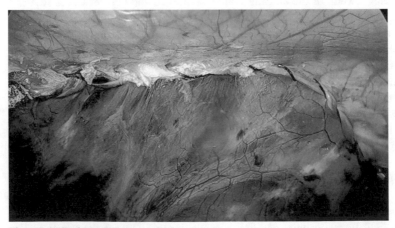

Fig. 11.20 Peritoneal closure completed

underlying structures of the landing zone by tissue penetration is to be avoided due to the risk of chronic pain. Larger hernias like PM3, PL3 still deserve improved retention by fibrin sealant or cyanoacrylate (CA) glue mesh fixation in order to prevent an early mesh dislocation (Fig. 11.18). The author's personal experience of 15 years and over 2000 meshes fixed with CA glue supported by the very low cost of the material does not allow refraining from the additional security offered by the adhesive fixation [11].

11.3.5 Peritoneal Closure

Meticulous running suture of the peritoneal flap prevents any contact of prosthetic with the intestinal loops and avoids any obstructive event based on incarceration or strangulation within a defect in an incomplete closure (Figs. 11.19 and 11.20).

11.3.6 Closure of the Trocar Incisions

The working ports of 10 mm or more can cause trocar hernias and therefore should be closed in layers [7].

11.4   The Advantage of the TAPP Technique

In TAPP the endoscope enters an existing space enlarged by CO_2 insufflation. The larger working space allows for a greater degree of movement and improves dexterity. The free view of the groin defect on the ipsilateral and contralateral side facilitates anatomic orientation, improves correctness of the preoperative diagnosis and helps to develop a clear operative strategy. The exploration of the abdominal cavity is possible. Looking behind the peritoneal flap is possible at any time. This increases dissectional safety in more complex situations.

In the author's opinion, TAPP has the widest range of indications. In primary and recurrent hernias, unilateral and bilateral, inguinal and femoral, in females and males, in elective and emergency settings, TAPP can be the technique of choice if expertise is present. The learning curve of TAPP is obviously shorter than that of TEP.

11.5   The Rationale of the TAPP Technique

The effectiveness of this repair is based on the mesh size and its placement. The importance of the surgeon's performance in terms of delicate and atraumatic dissection of the landing zone is crucial. The larger the mesh (accommodated in a very large landing zone) the lower the risk of recurrence. Non-penetrating fixation lowers the risk of postoperative chronic pain.

The laparoscopic approach to prosthetic hernia repair shows the lowest incidence of infections. In the author's personal experience, the infection rate of TAPP repair has been 0.0% over a period of 24 years.

11.6   The Logic of the TAPP Technique

Groin hernia is a very frequent occurrence to be electively treated. The advantages of a laparoscopic approach for the majority of intraabdominal pathologies are generally accepted. The necessary skills for these techniques have to be acquired, developed and trained in a frequent setting. The TAPP technique for hernia repair requires a wide spectrum of surgical gestures (including suturing) necessary for any advanced laparoscopic procedure.

In the author's personal opinion, the TAPP technique is easier to standardize, which makes teaching and learning easier. As this technique offers so many laparoscopic elements to be perfected in a very frequent procedure, it should become our ambition to make it to "the teaching operation" in order to become a logical part of a modern surgical curriculum. Thanks to the collective effort of many, guided by few (Simons, Miserez, Bittner, Bonjer), several milestone guidelines or consensus conferences on hernia repair were realized [7, 10, 12]. The technical aspects of TAPP repair were minutely worked out by Bittner [7, 10, 12–16] and Kukleta [7, 10–12, 16, 17] in order to facilitate structured teaching and to ease the learning curve of this useful procedure.

It often seems impossible ... until it's done
(Nelson Mandela)

References

1. Stoppa R, Petit J, Abourachid H (1973) Procédé original de plastie des hernies de l'aine: l'interposition sans fixation d'une prothèse en tulle de Dacron par voie médiane sous-péritonéal. Chirurgie 99:119–123
2. Fruchaud H (1956) Anatomie chirurgicale des hernies de l'aine. Doin, Paris
3. Arregui ME, Davis CJ, Yucel O, Nagan RF (1992) Laparoscopic mesh repair of inguinal hernia using a preperitoneal approach: a preliminary report. Surg Laparosc Endosc 2:53–58
4. DulucqJL (1991) Traitement des hernies de l'aine par mise en place d'un patch prothétique sous-péritonéal en rétro-péritonéoscopie. Cah Chir 79:15–16
5. Ferzli GS, Massad A, Albert P (1992) Extraperitoneal endoscopic inguinal hernia repair. J Laparoendosc Surg 2:281–286

6. McKernan JB, Laws HL (1993) Laparoscopic repair of inguinal hernias using a totally extraperitoneal prosthetic approach. Surg Endosc 7:26–28
7. Bittner R, Arregui ME, Bisgaard T et al (2011) Guidelines for laparoscopic (TAPP) and endoscopic (TEP) treatment of inguinal hernia (International Endohernia Society). Surg Endosc 25:2773–2843
8. Sakurai S (2015) Anatomy of groin. Shujutu 69:491–523 [Article in Japanese]
9. Sakurai S (2013) What is the space of Bogros, Retzius? The 9th International Congress of APHS 2013, Keynote Lecture
10. Simons MP, Aufenacker T, Bay-Nielsen M et al (2009) European Hernia Society guidelines on the treatment of inguinal hernia in adult patients. Hernia 13:343–403
11. Kukleta JF, Freytag C, Weber M (2012) Efficiency and safety of mesh fixation in laparoscopic inguinal hernia repair using n-butyl cyanoacrylate: long-term biocompatibility in over 1,300 mesh fixations. Hernia 16:152–162
12. Poelman MM, van den Heuvel B, Deelder JD et al (2013) EAES Consensus Development Conference on endoscopic repair of groin hernias. Surg Endosc 27:3505–3519
13. Bittner R, Sauerland S, Schmedt CG (2005) Comparison of endoscopic techniques vs Shouldice and other open nonmesh techniques for inguinal hernia repair: a meta-analysis of randomized controlled trials. Surg Endosc 19:605–615
14. Schmedt CG, Sauerland S, Bittner R (2005) Comparison of endoscopic procedures vs Lichtenstein and other open mesh techniques for inguinal hernia repair: a meta-analysis of randomized controlled trials. Surg Endosc 1:188–199
15. Leibl BJ, Jäger C, Kraft B et al (2005) Laparoscopic hernia repair–TAPP or/and TEP? Langenbecks Arch Surg 390:77–82
16. Bittner R, Montgomery A, Arregui ME et al (2015) Update of guidelines on laparoscopic (TAPP) and endoscopic (TEP) treatment of inguinal hernia (International Endohernia Society). Surg Endosc 29:289–321
17. Kukleta JF (2010) TAPP – The logic of hernia repair. Le Journal de Coelio-chirurgie 76:14–20

Total Extraperitoneal (TEP) Approach in Inguinal Hernia Repair: the Old and the New

12

Davide Lomanto and Eva Lourdes Sta. Clara

12.1 Introduction

Endoscopic inguinal hernia repair has three surgical approaches from totally extraperitoneal (TEP) repair to the transabdominal preperitoneal approach (TAPP) and the less common intraperitoneal onlay mesh repair (IPOM). The first two are widely utilized for the obvious advantages of lower recurrence and complication rates, and better outcome when compared to the open repair while covering the entire potential hernia site in the myopectineal orifice with a large prosthesis [1, 2].

There are some benefits related to each technique: overall, in the TEP approach there is minimal risk of intrabdominal injury to organs and postoperative adhesions, while in TAPP the contralateral side can be examined for an occult or undiagnosed hernia and it can be useful as a diagnostic tool in an emergency hernia repair or irreducible cases.

12.2 Indications

- Patient with primary or recurrent reducible inguinal hernia
- Fit for general anesthesia

D. Lomanto (✉)
Minimally Invasive Surgical Centre, Department of Surgery, YLL School of Medicine,
National University of Singapore
Singapore
e-mail: surdl@nus.edu.sg

G. Campanelli (Ed), *Inguinal Hernia Surgery*,
Updates in Surgery
DOI: 10.1007/978-88-470-3947-6_12, © Springer-Verlag Italia 2017

12.3   Contraindications

- Not fit for general anesthesia
- Acute abdomen with strangulated and infected bowel
- Respiratory distress
- Pediatric patients

12.4   Relative Contraindications

- Irreducible hernia
- Sliding hernia
- Inguinoscrotal hernia
- Previous prostatectomy or pelvic surgery
- Previous TEP/TAPP repair

Previous lower abdominal surgery is a relative contraindication. Adhesions can pose difficulty to the attending surgeon, thus a surgeon who is attempting this should be skilled in both TEP and the transabdominal preperitoneal approach. However, it should be explained to the patient that there is also a possibility that the operation may be converted to an open approach, as deemed necessary by the surgeon. Previous open appendectomies are usually not a problem but they require one to be more careful during the lateral dissection.

Recurrent hernia from a previous TEP is a relative contraindication. This can still be done through TEP depending on the expertise of the surgeon.

Large inguinoscrotal hernia is also a relative contraindication depending on the experience of the surgeon, since there would usually be a distorted anatomy and limited working space in this kind of inguinal hernias.

12.5   Preoperative Preparation

A thorough history and physical examination is necessary to assess the patient including fitness for general anesthesia. If there is any doubt in the diagnosis of the inguinal hernia (large defect, sliding hernia, multiple recurrent, etc.) it may be prudent to do a preoperative imaging work-up by dynamic ultrasound or CT scan.

It should also be explained to the patient that there might be a risk of conversion to transabdominal preperitoneal (TAPP) inguinal hernia repair or an open approach depending on the difficulty and safety of the procedure, which is based on the judgment of the attending surgeon. Risk for recurrence and complications should be properly explained to the patient including vascular, nerve and vas injury, seroma, mesh infection, postoperative chronic pain, etc. [3].

Prophylactic antibiotic treatment is recommended in the presence of risk factors for wound and mesh infection based on patient status (advanced age, recurrent corticosteroid use, immunosuppressive conditions, obesity, diabetes, and malignancy) or surgical factors (contamination, long operation duration, use of drains, urinary catheter) [4, 5].

Patients should also be advised to void prior to the procedure.

However, in the case of complicated hernias (partially reducible, large defect) and/or length of surgery more than 1.5 hrs it is advisable to decompress the urinary bladder by inserting a urinary catheter which can be removed at the end of the procedure.

12.6 Operating Theatre Setup

12.6.1 Instruments

- 10 or 5 mm, 30-degree angled telescopes
- Trocars
  - (1) 10-mm Hasson's trocar
  - (2) 5-mm trocar
- Balloon dissector
  Based on the IEHS guidelines, it is recommended to use a balloon dissector when creating the preperitoneal space, especially during the learning period, when it is difficult to identify the correct preperitoneal plane and space. Once the learning curve is overcome, to reduce the cost of the procedure, a blind dissection can be achieved by swiping the telescope along the midline. A self-made dissector balloon can be arranged using finger gloves over an irrigation device.
- Graspers and atraumatic graspers
- Scissors
- Prosthetic mesh
  It is advisable to use a large-pore polypropylene or multifilament polyester mesh with a size of at least 10 × 15 cm. Using a smaller mesh will increase the risk of recurrence. However, for larger defects of more than 3-4 cm (L >3 according to EHS classification [4, 5]) it is recommended to use a larger mesh (12 × 17 cm).
- Tackers and fixation devices
  According to the IEHS Guidelines and EBM, fixation of the mesh is required only in particular cases like large hernia defect (>3-4 cm), especially if direct, to avoid translation of the mesh and to reduce the risk of recurrence. Today either absorbable or permanent staplers/tackers are utilized to fix the mesh to Cooper's ligament and to the rectus muscle. Sealants in the form of fibrin glue

(Tisseel or Tissucol, Baxter USA) or synthetic glue (Liquiband, AMS UK; Histoacryl, BBraun, Germany, etc.) are also available and several studies have shown their efficacy and benefits.

- Endoloops
  Pre-made loop sutures are useful for closure of inadvertent tears in the peritoneum and ligation of the hernia sac. Based on the IEHS guidelines, it is recommended to close any peritoneal tears to decrease the risk of adhesions which may lead to bowel obstruction. If not commercially available, the loop can be made using a 50-70-cm absorbable suture and an extracorporeal Roeder knot.

12.6.2   Patient and Surgical Team Positioning

The patient lies supine in a slight Trendelenberg position (10-15 degrees) with both arms tucked at the sides, under general anesthesia. The attending surgeon stands on the side opposite the hernia defect side and the assistant stands beside the attending surgeon at the cephalad side of the patient (Fig. 12.1). The nurse stands on the same side as the surgeon, near the feet of the patient. The monitor and video equipment are placed at the caudal end of the operating table, either midline or slightly ipsilateral to the defect. Monitors mounted on a Boom arm will be helpful in improving visual space.

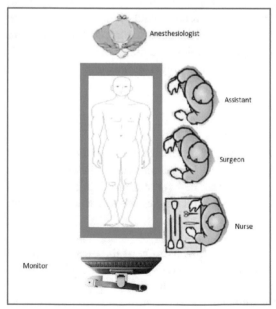

Fig. 12.1 Operating room set-up

12.7   Surgical Technique

12.7.1   Entering and creating the Preperitoneal Space

There are few techniques to enter and create the preperitoneal space. A 10-mm vertical infraumbilical incision is first made. Subcutaneous tissue is bluntly dissected to expose the anterior rectus sheath using (2) S-retractors (Fig. 12.2). The anterior rectus sheath is then incised, lateral from the midline, on the ipsilateral side of the hernia. This will avoid the linea alba and accidentally entering the peritoneal cavity. Then the rectus muscle is retracted laterally to expose the posterior rectus sheath (Fig. 12.3).

Once the preperitoneal plane is entered, there are a few techniques to create the space: 1. the optical ballon dissector; 2. the Veress' needle technique; 3. the

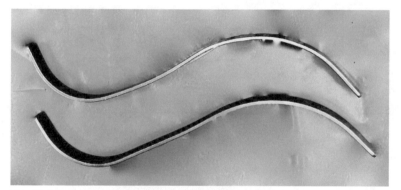

Fig. 12.2 Anterior rectus sheath exposed using S-retractors

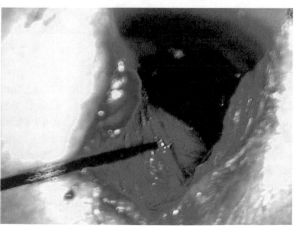

Fig. 12.3 Rectus muscle retracted laterally

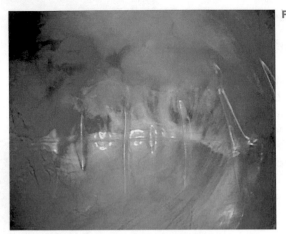

Fig. 12.4 Balloon dissector

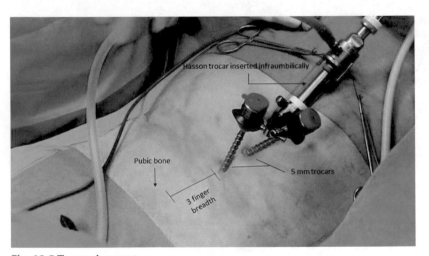

Fig. 12.5 Trocar placement

most common blunt dissection. Using the trocar with an optical ballon dissector, the space is created by inflating the balloon under vision (Fig. 12.4). This is the plane one should maintain and create up to the symphysis pubis using a gauze, finger or a dissecting balloon, depending on the preference and expertise of the surgeon. A Hasson's trocar is then inserted and the plane is confirmed by inserting a 30-degree trocar. The rectus muscle should be visualized in the anterior area to be in the right plane. Insufflation is done with carbon dioxide at 8-12 mmHg.

Two 5-mm trocars are then inserted at the midline under direct vision to prevent any injury to the bladder, peritoneum, or bowels. The first 5-mm trocar is placed 3 finger breadths above the symphysis pubis. The second 5-mm trocar is then placed in between the Hasson's trocar and the first 5-mm trocar (Fig 12.5).

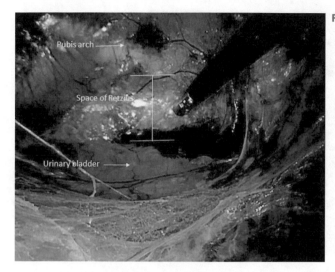

Fig. 12.6 Space of Retzius

12.7.2   Medial Dissection (Space of Retzius or Prevesical Space)

Once all the working ports are inserted, using two atraumatic graspers, the dissection is conducted along the midline, below the rectus muscle and towards the pubis arch. The dissection should go 2 cm beyond the symphysis pubis to the obturator fossa to avoid missing any obturator hernia and to allow the medial lower corner of the mesh to be fixated once the space is deflated (Fig. 12.6). The limits of the dissection are: medially, 1-2 cm beyond the midline and below the pubis arch; inferiorly until the peritoneal reflection is identified at the border with the retroperitoneal space.

12.7.3   Lateral Dissection (Lateral Space of Bogros)

Moving towards the anterior superior iliac spine (ASIS), in a surgical plane that is below the inferior epigastric vessels (IEV) and above the peritoneum, the lateral dissection is made. This plane is confined by the two layers of the fascia transversalis. The dissection is continued by pushing down the peritoneum until the psoas muscle can be seen. The lateral space of Bogros is delineated and cleaned all the way up to the anterior superior iliac spine. Attention should be made to avoid dissecting further laterally, beyond the lumbar fascia in the so-called "lateral triangle of pain". This will prevent injury to the latero-cutaneous and genitofemoral nerves. The thin layer of fat covering the lateral fascia should be preserved and not skeletonized; similarly, energy and diathermy should not be used at this level. (Figs. 12.7 and 12.8). The limits of the lateral dissection are inferiorly the psoas muscle, superiorly the ASIS and cranially the arcuate line.

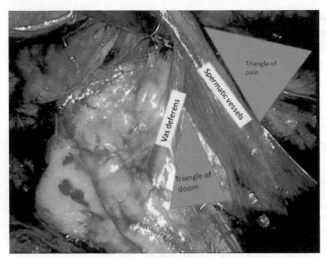

Fig. 12.7 Triangle of pain and triangle of doom

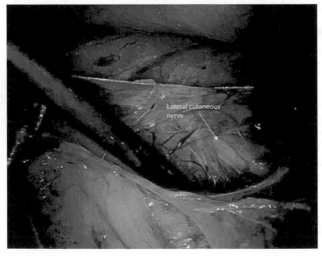

Fig. 12.8 Lateral cutaneous nerve at the space of Bogros

12.7.4 Hernia Sac Identification and Reduction

Once the medial and lateral dissection is completed (Fig. 12.9), we should be able to identify the entire hernia defect, followed by a proper hernia sac reduction and repair. This will allow the surgeon to visualize all the anatomical landmarks, to lessen the risk of injuries, to have a wider space for placing the prosthesis and, in case of inadvertent tear of the peritoneum, to continue to work safely without being affected by the pneumoperitoneum.

Exposure of the whole myopectineal orifice should be made after a complete medial and lateral dissection followed by the hernia sac reduction (Fig. 12.10).

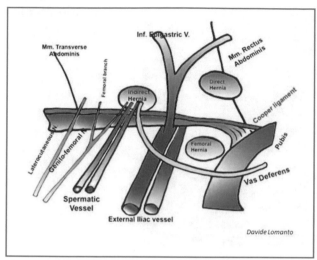

Fig. 12.9 Anatomic landmarks in endo-laparoscopic inguinal hernia repair

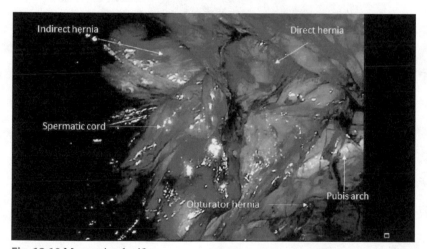

Fig. 12.10 Myopectineal orifice

12.7.5 Hernia Reduction

Medial or Direct Hernia In the endolaparoscopic approach, a defect medial to the inferior epigastric hernia and at the level of the Hesselbach's triangle is a direct hernia. Reduction can be easily achieved by identifying and holding the hernia "pseudosac" and dividing it from the preperitoneal lipoma and peritoneum. Special care should be taken once the pubis arch is reached because of the risk of injury to the "corona mortis" and laterally to the iliac vessels and vas deferens. The "pseudosac" is grabbed and the hernia contents are then reduced.

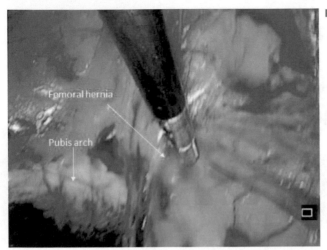

Fig. 12.11 Femoral hernia

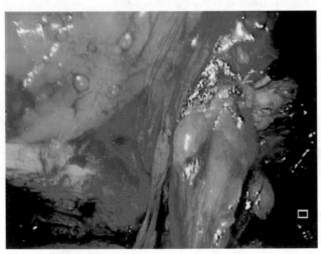

Fig. 12.12 Widening of the femoral ring at the medial-upper side

Femoral Hernia Reduction of the hernia sac and content is achieved by gentle traction keeping in mind that the vessels hide behind the content (Fig. 12.11). If the content is not reducible by traction due to the small size of the defect, it may be necessary to widen the femoral defect by using a hook diathermy ONLY on the medial-upper side (Fig. 12.12). This will facilitate the hernia sac reduction.

Obturator Hernia In the same canal where the obturator vessels are, it is possible that a preperitoneal fat and/or hernia sac is within. As in femoral hernia, a gentle traction will allow the reduction of the hernia sac (Fig. 12.13).

Indirect Hernia Lateral to the IEV lies the deep ring and indirect hernia. The standard approach to indirect hernia repair requires the spermatic structures to be separated from the hernia sac. This can be achieved using the medial approach and

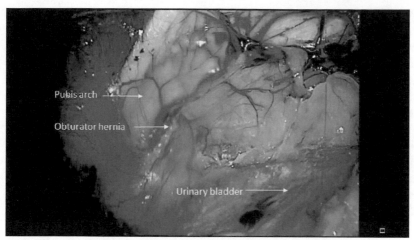

Fig. 12.13 Obturator hernia

four simple steps: 1. Separating the whole sac and spermatic cord from the iliac vessels; 2. Slimming the sac at the level of the deep ring with a partial reduction of both cord structures and sac; 3. Separating the cord structures from the sac on the inferior edge of the sac; 4. Reducing the sac by simple traction or transection. This can be necessary in cases of long or complete sac in order to minimize injury to the testis by overtraction. It is suggested to divide the sac using diathermy to reduce the risk of hematoma and to ligate the proximal part using pre-made suture loops. Lipoma of the cord should be fully reduced.

It is important to close all peritoneal holes/tears with absorbable suture loops or plastic clips (i.e., hem-o-lok, Teleflex Medical, USA) to prevent any internal herniation or adhesion formation with the mesh. Once reduced or ligated, the peritoneal sac should be further reduced until the peritoneal reflection is visualized and medially separated by the adhesion with the vas deferens.

12.7.6 Mesh Repair

The final step is the hernia repair, which is achieved by covering the entire myopectineal orifice with a synthetic large-pore prosthesis of 10 × 15 cm. The mesh is rolled up and inserted through the 10-mm trocar. A "no-touch technique" is mandatory to avoid mesh infection. The mesh is opened and inserted into the preperitoneal cavity avoiding any contact with the skin. The mesh is then placed horizontally and unrolled over the myopectineal orifice making sure to cover all the hernia sites. One-third of the mesh should be below the symphysis pubis, the upper margin reaching the lower trocar medially and laterally lying over the psoas muscle. In bilateral hernias, there should be a 1-2-cm overlap of the meshes at the midline. It is important to make sure that no part of the peritoneum is under the mesh to prevent any recurrence.

The mesh is then anchored using tackers or sealant to prevent mesh migration and possible recurrence. Two to three points of fixation are necessary: Cooper's ligament, medial to the inferior epigastric vessels at the rectus muscle and, if necessary, lateral to the inferior epigastric vessels. Avoid tacker or stapler fixation below the iliopubic tract and too laterally considering 15-20% of abnormalities in the nerve paths. This will help to prevent any nerve injuries and consequent postoperative chronic pain.

An accurate hemostasis should be guaranteed if the correct surgical plane is identified. The carbon dioxide is then released while checking visually that the mesh is not rolled and the peritoneum stays in front of the mesh so as to prevent any recurrence. The lateral inferior edge of the mesh can be held with a grasper, if necessary. The ports are then removed and the anterior rectus sheath incision at the 10-mm trocar site is sutured. The skin incisions are then closed with absorbable sutures or glue.

12.8   Reduced and Single Port Technique

Since the advent of the laparoscopic technique the trend towards scarless surgical techniques continued. Since then, a few novel approaches have been utilized in hernia repair such as needlescopic surgery and the single incision endolaparoscopic surgery (SPES) [6, 7].

For needlescopic surgery, smaller-size instrumentation is utilized to perform the procedure, challenges are the flexibility of the instruments especially in large defects or thickened peritonal sac. Clinical studies showed comparable results with the standard technique but nevertheless the needlescopic technique has never been successful with worldwide acceptance [6, 8].

The latest approach, SPES, which uses a single device in which all the telescope and working ports are inserted, has seen much enthusiasm not only for inguinal hernia repair but for also cholecystectomy, appendectomy, adrenalectomy, etc. [9–13]. The possible advantages of single or reduced port surgery in hernia repair can be attributed to less pain, better cosmesis, less risk for port-site hernia, and even shorter hospital stays. A technical challenge is the ergonomics, as the approach is more affected by constraints in exposure, adequate retraction, conflict between the instruments, and lack of triangulation [14]. In standard TEP with a midline approach, this is less evident because of the almost parallel axis of the two working ports, resulting in a shorter learning curve.

Recent studies also show at least equivalent pain scores, operative duration and complication rates when comparing conventional laparoscopic surgery to reduced/single port surgery in hernia repair, making this novel approach acceptable and comparable to standard TEP inguinal hernia repair [15, 16].

12.9   Postoperative Care

- Diet as tolerated is resumed
- Analgesics are given (etoricoxib 90 mg daily for 3 days)
- Patient is discharged on the same day once voiding freely
- Follow-up is at 1 week, 1 and 3 months

12.10   Complications

Complications can be categorized into intraoperative and postoperative complications. Intraoperative complications specific to TEP occur in about 4-6% of the cases and can be due to injury to vascular, visceral, nerve and spermatic cord structures [17–19]. Vascular injuries would include injury to the external iliac vessels, inferior epigastric vessels, spermatic vessels or the vessels over the pubic arch including the corona mortis veins. The most common are injury to the IEV and this can be avoided by using the midline approach and by inserting all the ports under direct vision. Injury to the major vessels is catastrophic, a correct lateral traction of the sac and spermatic structure with medial approach may be helpful in avoiding it. A careful practice should be used when retracting or dissecting closer to the "triangle of doom". Visceral injuries including but not limited to the bowels and urinary tract can be reduced by careful dissection and limiting the use of diathermy. Transmitted energy through the thin peritoneal layer may result in injury to the underlying bowel. Patients with previous pelvis surgey, sliding hernia, large inguinoscrotal hernia are at risk for bladder injury, in which case urinary catheterization may be necessary. In the event of injuries, these can be managed by an endolaparoscopoic suture repair. Nerve injuries can be prevented by accurate lateral dissection, limiting the number of staplers/tackers if fixation is needed, and using of absorbable tackers or sealant. Spermatic cord injuries can be lessened by properly identifying the anatomy and avoiding too much traction of the cord. Tears in the peritoneum can also occur especially during the early stage of the learning curve. All peritoneal tears should be closed by using suture loops or hem-o-loks.

Postoperative complications like seroma commonly occur in patients with large direct and indirect hernias. The seroma usually appears after 7-10 days and does not require any treatment. It may be mistaken for an early recurrence. In principle, it should be treated conservatively, and will be reabsorbed spontaneously within 4-6 weeks. However, if it is symptomatic and persisting after 2 months it is advisable to drain it by aspiration and in sterile condition. In the case of complex sero-hematoma an excision after 4-5 months can be necessary.

Early recurrence is usually due to inadequate surgical technique and can be due to wrong case selection for beginners, inadequate fixation of the mesh, inadequate mesh size, inadequate dissection of the myopectineal orifice and failure to cover unidentified hernia defects [20].

12.11   Conclusions

Several clinical trials and meta-analyses have shown endoscopic preperitoneal hernia repair (TEP) performed by experienced surgeons to be associated with reduced postoperative pain, less need for postoperative analgesia, earlier return to work, fewer complications and a low recurence rate when compared to open mesh repair [1, 2, 21, 22]. These benefits will be more significant if the laparoscopic treatment is for bilateral or recurrent hernias. As for any successful surgical technique – but especially in hernia repair – a careful patient selection, a good understanding of the anatomy, an adequate surgical technique and the surgeon's experience are very important key factors to achieve a good clinical outcome with a low rate of short-term and long-term complications.

References

1. Memon MA, Cooper NJ, Memon B et al (2003) Meta-analysis of randomized clinical trials comparing open and laparoscopic inguinal hernia repair. Br J Surg 90:1479–1492
2. Feliu X, Claveria R, Besora P et al (2011) Bilateral inguinal hernia repair: laparoscopic or open approach? Hernia 15:15–18
3. Lomanto D, Katara AN (2006) Managing intraoperative complications during totally extraperitoneal repair of inguinal hernia. Minim Access Surg 2:165–170
4. Simons MP, Aufenacaker T, Bay-Nielsen M et al (2009) European Hernia Society guidelines on the treatment of inguinal hernia in adult patients. Hernia 13:343–403
5. Bittner R, Arregui ME, Bisgaard T et al (2011) Guidelines for laparoscopic (TAPP) and endoscopic (TEP) treatment of inguinal hernia [International EndoHernia Society (IEHS)]. Surg Endosc 25:2773–2843
6. Goo TT, Lawenko M, Cheah WK, Lomanto D (2010) Endoscopic total extraperitoneal repair of recurrent inguinal hernia: a 5-year review. Hernia 14:477–480
7. Lau H, Lee F (2002) A prospective comparative study of needlescopic and conventional endoscopic TEP hernioplasty. Surg Endosc 16:1737–1740
8. Goo TT, Goel R, Lawenko M, Lomanto D (2010) Laparoscopic transabdominal preperitoneal (TAPP) hernia repair via a single port. Surg Laparosc Endosc Percutan Tech 20:389–390
9. Wada H, Kimura T, Kawabe A et al (2012) Laparoscopic TAPP inguinal hernia repair using needlescopic instruments: a 15-year single centre experience in 317 patients. Surg Endosc 26:1898–1902
10. Trastulli S, Cirocchi R, Desiderio J et al (2013) Systematic review and meta-analysis of randomized clinical trials comparing single-incision versus conventional laparoscopic cholecystectomy. Br J Surg 100:191–208
11. Fung AK, Aly EH (2012) Systematic review of single incision laparoscopic colonic surgery. Br J Surg 99:1353–1364
12. Rehman H, Mathews T, Ahmed I (2012) A review of minimally invasive single port/incision laparoscopic appendectomy. J Laparoendosc Adv Surg Tech 22:641–646
13. Goo TT, Agarwal A, Goel R et al (2011) Single-port access adrenalectomy: our initial experience. J Laparoendosc Adv Surg Tech A 21:815–819
14. Goel R Lomanto D (2012) Controversies in single port surgery. Surg Laparosc Endosc Percutan Tech 22:380–382
15. Fuentes MB, Goel R, Lee-Ong AC et al (2013) Single-port endo-laparoscopic surgery (SPES) for totally extraperitoneal inguinal hernia: a critical appraisal of the chopstick repair. Hernia 17:217–221

16. Wijerathne S, Agarwal N, Ramzy A et al (2016) Single-port versus conventional laparoscopic total extra-peritoneal inguinal hernia repair: a prospective, randomized, controlled clinical trial. Surg Endosc 30:1356–1363
17. Tetik C, Arregui ME, Dulucq JL et al (1994) Complications and recurrences with laparoscopic repair of groin hernias. A multi-institutional retrospective analysis. Surg Endosc 8:1316–1323
18. Kraus MA (1993) Nerve injury during laparoscopic inguinal hernia repair. Surg Laparosc Endosc 3:342–345
19. Felix E, Habertson N, Varteian S (1999) Laparoscopic hernioplasty: surgical complications. Surg Endosc 13:328–331
20. Miguel PR, Reusch M, daRosa AL, Carlos JR (1998) Laparoscopic hernia repair – complications. JSLS 2:35–40
21. Cavazzola LT, Rosen MJ (2013) Laparoscopic versus open inguinal hernia repair. Surg Clin North Am 93:1269–1279
22. Bittner R, Montgomery MA, Arregui E et al (2015) Update of guidelines on laparoscopic (TAPP) and endoscopic (TEP) treatment of inguinal hernia (International Endohernia Society). Surg Endosc 29:289–321

Robotic Transabdominal Preperitoneal Inguinal Hernia Repair

13

Conrad D. Ballecer, Edward L. Felix, and Brian E. Prebil

13.1   Introduction

While the DaVinci robot (Intuitive Surgical Inc.) has been in use since the turn of the century, its application and adoption in the field of general surgery has been slow. Barriers to adoption of the robotic platform include, but are not limited to, concerns of cost, a general fear of new innovation, and a paucity of data demonstrating value relative to conventional laparoscopy. Despite the above, robotic technology has recently experienced a rapid growth in the field of general surgery in the United States. Its exponential growth in large part can be attributed to its adoption in the hernia space for both minimally invasive surgical (MIS) repairs of ventral and inguinal hernias (Figs. 13.1 and 13.2). Adoption can be explained by many factors such as improved ergonomics, precision, and visualization which many believe translates into an enabling or facilitating technology.

Surgeons who regularly offer laparoscopy for inguinal hernia repair comprise an overwhelming minority despite its well established benefits. Adoption rates vary from 14 to 19% in the United States. Many attribute low penetration rates as a testament to the difficulty of the approach, which requires both a comprehensive understanding of the anatomy of Fruchaud's myopectineal orifice (MPO) as well as the technical skill to surgically intervene within this space. The proposed enabling effect of the robotic instrument has allowed many surgeons to regularly incorporate MIS hernia repair into their practice. This statement underscores a very important concept in that robotic inguinal hernia repair should be considered analogous to the laparoscopic approach performed with a different instrument and as such, well-established principles of posterior hernia repair must be adhered to.

C.D. Ballecer (✉)
Center for Minimally Invasive and Robotic Surgery
Peoria, Arizona, USA
e-mail: cballecer@cmirs.com

G. Campanelli (Ed), *Inguinal Hernia Surgery,*
Updates in Surgery
DOI: 10.1007/978-88-470-3947-6_13, © Springer-Verlag Italia 2017

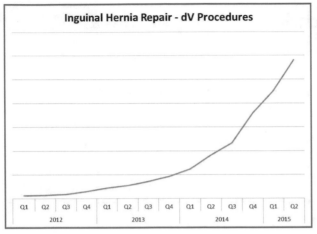

Fig. 13.1 Adoption of robotic inguinal hernia repair (courtesy of Intuitive Surgical Inc.)

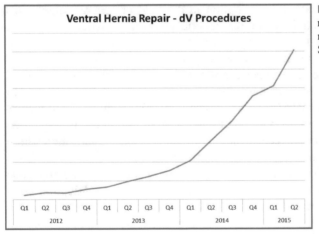

Fig. 13.2 Adoption of robotic ventral hernia repair (courtesy of Intuitive Surgical Inc.)

This chapter is dedicated to detailing the robotic transabdominal preperitoneal inguinal hernia repair (r-TAPP) technique implicitly adhering to the principles well established in conventional laparoscopy.

13.2 Patient Positioning, Trocar Set-up, Docking, and Instrumentation

The patient can either be placed in a conventional supine or lithotomy position. Port position and trocar set-up is analogous to that of traditional laparoscopic repair (Fig. 13.3). We prefer open supraumbilical entry with a 12-mm balloon trocar although an 8.5-mm daVinci (dV) trocar for the 8-mm camera may also be

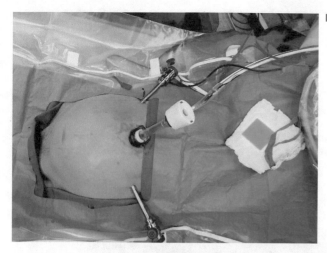

Fig. 13.3 Port position

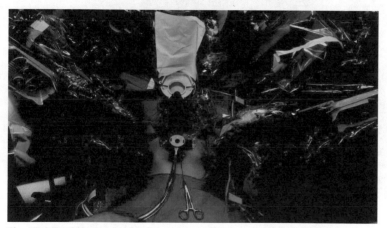

Fig. 13.4 Docking in a supine lithotomy position

utilized. Either 5-mm or 8-mm instrument trocars are then placed 10 cm lateral to the camera port, irrespective of the site of the hernia.

While there are many options to dock the robot, we prefer docking in between the legs with the patient in a supine lithotomy position (Fig. 13.4). Docking over either hip, however, can also be employed which will achieve equal access to both right and left groins in the setting of bilateral hernias.

For most cases we utilize two instruments including the dV prograsp and dV monopolar scissors (Fig. 13.5). With this instrumentation profile, we also use an absorbable tacker to fixate and reperitonealize the mesh. A suture-cut needle driver can also be used for blunt dissection as well as suture mesh fixation and re-approximation of the peritoneal defect. For patients with large inguinoscrotal hernias, a dV Maryland bipolar grasper may be considered helpful to facilitated hernia sac reduction.

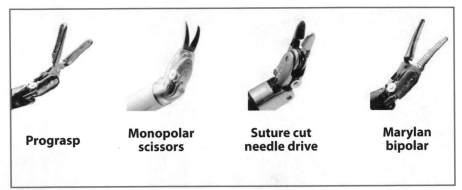

| **Prograsp** | **Monopolar scissors** | **Suture cut needle drive** | **Marylan bipolar** |

Fig. 13.5 dV Instrumentation

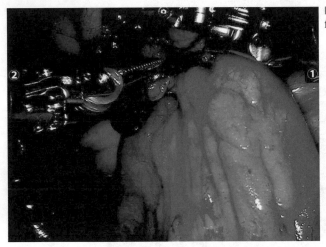

Fig. 13.6 Incarcerated femoral hernia

We prefer the use of a 12-mm zero-degree scope although this is also optional at the operator's discretion. After docking of the robot, the instruments are placed under direct vision.

13.3   Technical Steps

13.3.1   Reduction of the Hernia Content

As in any hernia repair, the first part of the procedure involves reduction of the hernia content. Incarcerated bowel contents through an inguinofemoral hernia must be dealt with safely and meticulously (Fig. 13.6). When aggressive bowel handling is required, the dV fenestrated bipolar instrument is used because of its lower grip strength in comparison to the dV prograsp.

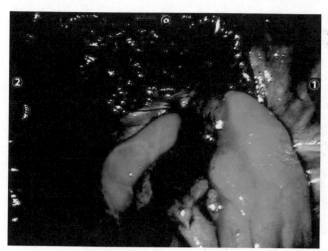

Fig. 13.7 Firefly assessment of bowel viability

In the setting of incarcerated bowel contents and following successful reduction, viability of the intestinal segment must be assured. We routinely employ Firefly technology as an adjunctive measure to assess intestinal perfusion (Fig. 13.7). This technology is similar to the use of fluorescein and a Wood's lamp to evaluate bowel viability. Five ml of indocyanine-green (IcG) is administered and intestinal perfusion can be assessed within a minute of injection. The bowel is confirmed to be viable if under Firefly view it demonstrates a green tone.

A strangulated segment of bowel mandates bowel resection which may affect definitive repair. In our practice, definitive repair with mesh is deferred in the setting of bowel resection for strangulated hernias. A peritoneal patch is sutured over the defect to minimize the risk of immediate recurrence.

13.3.2   Evaluation of the Surface Anatomy

After successful reduction of the hernia content, key surface anatomical landmarks are identified (Fig. 13.8). Accurate identification of key landmarks will not only delineate the type of hernia present, but also provides a road map to guide preperitoneal dissection. The bedside assistant is advised to palpate the level of the anterior superior iliac spine (ASIS) to reference the position of the iliopubic tract. This will also help determine the site of initial peritoneal incision.

13.3.3   Peritoneal Incision

A high peritoneal tranverse incision is made from the level well above ASIS to the level of the median umbilical ligament. This transverse incision should be made a minimum of 5 cm cephalad to the superior aspect of the hernia defect. This

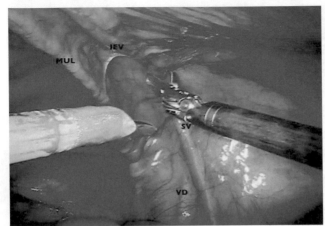

Fig. 13.8 Surface anatomy (*MUL*, medial umbilical ligament; *IEV*, inferior epigastric vessels; *VD*, vas deferens; *SV*, spermatic vessels)

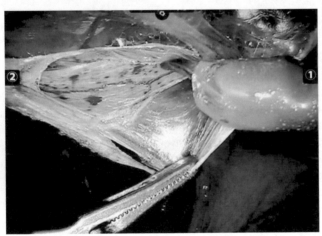

Fig. 13.9 Preperitoneal dissection

allows for both adequate cephalad overlap of the mesh and creating a redundancy in the peritoneal flap to facilitate reperitonealization of the mesh. It is common to include the transversalis fascia within the initial incision but every attempt is made to initiate flap dissection in the true preperitoneal space (Fig. 13.9). True preperitoneal dissection orients the operator within the correct plane for hernia sac reduction and final flap development. Benefits of exploiting this space also include avoidance of perforating vessels to the the overlying rectus muscle which can cause unnecessary bleeding. The true preperitoneal space is avascular allowing for blunt dissection to the level of the hernia sac. Given the translucency of the peritoneum within the correct plane, meticulous dissection is required to avoid creating peritoneal rents and tears. A consistent awareness of visual stimuli or cues is employed to overcome the loss of haptic feedback during peritoneal retraction and manipulation.

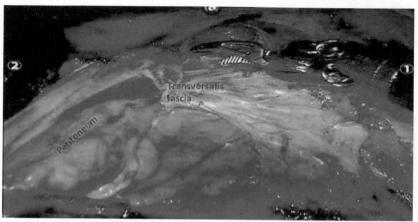

Fig. 13.10 Hernia sac reduction

13.3.4 Hernia Sac Reduction

All attempts are made to follow the peritoneum to insure proper plane dissection. Direct hernia sacs occurring medial to the epigastric vessels and above the iliopubic tract tend to reduce readily. The peritoneal sac is dissected free from the transversalis fascia (Fig. 13.10). In the setting of an indirect sac, medial and lateral dissection is performed to isolate the peritoneal invagination. Meticulous dissection of the peritoneum from the cord structures or female equivalents is required employing only judicious use of cautery to avoid bleeding and unintentional injury to nerves which can lead to chronic pain. Primarily blunt dissection is performed to dissect the peritoneum off the vas deferens and spermatic vessels. In the setting of large inguinoscrotals, the sac can be transected with the distal sac left in situ; however, we prefer to completely reduce the sac intact and invert back into the intraperitoneal cavity. We routinely divide the round ligament in females to facilitate peritoneal dissection. It is mandatory to reduce cord lipomas out of the deep inguinal ring which are then resected or left in situ, provided they do not interrupt the subsequent placement of mesh.

13.3.5 Critical View of the Myopectineal Orifice

While the critical view of safety for gallbladder surgery is a well-established and accepted mandate, the critical view of the myopectineal orifice is not as well known. According to the rule of laparoscopic cholecystectomy, no clips should be placed prior to achieving the critical view. Similarly, we believe that mesh should not be placed prior to obtaining the critical view of the myopectineal orifice.

Medial Dissection Dissection medial to the inferior epigastric vessels should expose and demonstrate the direct space, the femoral canal, and the obturator foramina (Figs. 13.11 and 13.12). Dissection of Cooper's ligament should extend

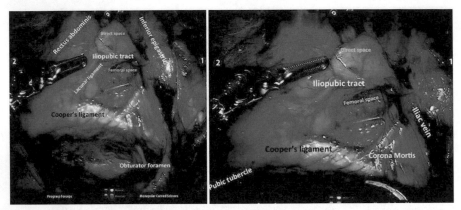

Fig. 13.11 Medial dissection

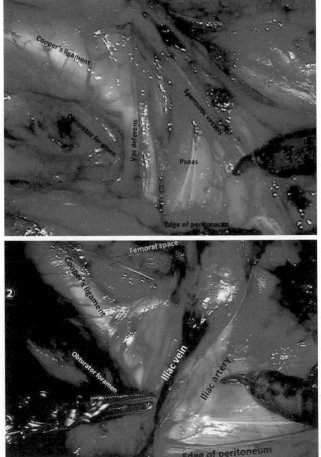

Fig. 13.12 Cord dissection

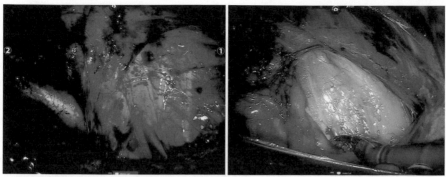

Fig. 13.13 Lateral dissection

across the midline isolating the pubis; below which is the space of Retzius exposed by blunt dissection of the bladder off the pubic bone.

Cord Dissection The peritoneal sac is reduced and the cord structures or the female equivalents are parietalized. This requires adequate posterior peritoneal dissection which will minimize the incidence of peritoneum sneaking under the inferior edge of the mesh leading to a common cause of recurrence after MIS inguinal hernia repair. This requires meticulous dissection to avoid injury to the cord structures and sensory nerves, injury to which may lead to testicular ischemia and chronic pain. With adequate posterior peritoneal dissection, the triangle of doom will be well delineated (Fig. 13.12) Careful dissection within the right plane is also mandatory to avoid major vascular injury to the iliac vessels.

Lateral Dissection Lateral dissection of the myopectineal orifice is mandatory to allow for the placement of a large mesh which adequately overlaps all four potential spaces: indirect space, direct space, femoral space, and obturator foramina. The extent of posterior peritoneal dissection should be confluent from the space of Retzius to the level of the ASIS. Within this territory resides the triangle of doom, site of critical sensory nerves which must be preserved to minimize the risk of chronic pain (Fig. 13.13).

13.3.6 Mesh Placement and Fixation

It is our philosophy that a large (10 × 15 cm at minimum) mesh should be placed that accepts the contours of the MPO. We use a 12 × 15 sheet of flat mesh, and will occasionally go larger for big direct hernias.

There are a myriad of options for both introducing and fixating the mesh flat to cover the MPO. Mesh and suture can be introduced prior to peritoneal dissection or once dissection is complete. Flat mesh can generally be introduced through the 8.5-mm trocars. We place our mesh after dissection is complete (Fig. 13.14). The robotic arm ipsilateral to the hernia defect is undocked and mesh is introduced by the bedside assistant via the ipsilateral trocar and directed to the pubic bone.

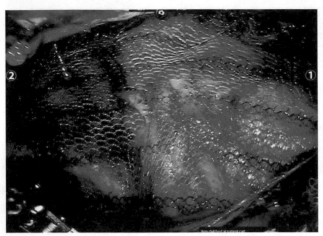

Fig. 13.14 Mesh placement

Coordination between the operator and the bedside assistant is required to lay the mesh flat with adequate coverage of all potential spaces. Alternatively, the trocar can be re-docked and the operator can lay the mesh in a correct position utilizing two grasping instruments. Prior to fixation, mesh placement is tested by manipulating the peritoneum to insure the mesh does not fold or buckle, with particular attention paid to the inferior edge of the mesh.

According to surgeon preference and mesh choice, there are options for no fixation, fixation with glue, sutures, or tacks. We have utilized all four options in our practice. Generally, we fixate the mesh with absorbable tacks: one tack on Cooper's ligament, one tack high superomedial, and one tack high superolateral. The latter two placed well above the iliopubic tract to avoid nerve entrapment. Intracorporeal suture fixation can also be performed in a similar fashion. Mechanical fixation is never employed below the iliopubic tract (save for Cooper's ligament), within the triangle of doom, nor the triangle of pain so as to avoid major vascular and nerve injury, respectively.

13.3.7   Reperitonealization of the Mesh

The peritoneal flap can be re-approximated to completely cover the mesh with either tacks or running suture (Fig. 13.15). If manipulation of the peritoneum causes buckling of the mesh, further posterior peritoneal dissection is advised. Significant gaps in the closure should be avoided to minimize the risk of early postoperative small bowel obstruction. Generally speaking, adequate peritoneal flap dissection will create a redundancy of the peritoneum allowing for tension-free re-approximation. The hernia sac can be used to obliterate any peritoneal rents. Alternatively, sutures can be used to close small peritoneal tears.

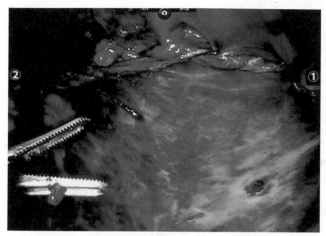

Fig. 13.15 Reperitonealization of mesh

13.3.8 The 10 Commandments of Felix

Edward Felix is well regarded as one of the pioneers of laparoscopic inguinal hernia repair, expert in both laparoscopic transabdominal and totally extraperitoneal approaches. Below he lists his 10 commandments which applies to all the different approaches for the repair of inguinal hernias via the posterior approach. It has served as a guide for our practice in successfully executing an inherently difficult operation with the goal of minimizing recurrence and incidence of postoperative chronic pain.

1. Must not deviate from the basic principles of posterior hernia repair whether a TAPP, TEP, e-TEP (extended-view TEP) or r-TAPP is performed.
2. Must see and dissect the entire wall including the pubis across the midline to expose all four potential hernia spaces in every patient. Must avoid a missed hernia, an important cause of recurrence. The advantage of a laparoscopic repair is that it repairs and reinforces all four potential sites in every patient.
3. Must extend the mesh below the pubis, between the pubis and the bladder to prevent the bladder from lifting up the mesh as the bladder fills.
4. Must be able to see the iliac vein in order to prevent missing a femoral hernia. If the location of the iliac vein is obscured by tissue extending down from the peritoneum, there is a femoral hernia.
5. Must look for and dissect the tissue lateral to the vas and vessels, the lipoma. The lipoma must be pulled out of the internal ring in every patient. The lipoma can appear tiny, but may be the tip of the iceberg. Place it on top of the mesh at the end of the procedure. The lipoma does not need to be resected as long as its vasculature is maintained.
6. Must dissect laterally and inferiorly far enough so that the re-expanding peritoneum doesn't lift the mesh. In TEP or e-TEP watch the peritoneum cover the mesh. If the peritoneum lifts the mesh, start over.

7. Must dissect between the vas and vessels to prevent missing the tail of the indirect sac. Peritoneum under the mesh will lead to recurrence in the future.
8. Must use a large enough mesh to widely cover all four spaces and the pubis.
9. Completely and safely cover the entire mesh without leaving holes or gaps. Blind tacking to close the peritoneum should be avoided.
10. Must pick the inguinal hernia repair that is the best fit for the patient.

13.4   Conclusions

The emergence and exponential adoption of r-TAPP inguinal hernia repair in general surgery underscores the importance that this approach be treated as analogous to that of conventional laparoscopic TAPP inguinal hernia repair. Both are MIS approaches to the treatment of groin hernias that require a comprehensive understanding of the anatomy of the myopectineal orifice. Moreover, a high degree of advanced skill is also required in order to execute and adhere to the well established and studied principles based on both open and MIS experience. An MIS approach with the singular goal of minimizing recurrence rates and the incidence of postoperative chronic pain. The learning curve, therefore, must be respected. It is the goal of the authors to use this chapter as a guide to pave a surgeon's path through and well beyond this curve.

Suggested Readings

Escobar Dominguez JE, Ramos MG, Seetharamaiah R et al (2015) Feasibility of robotic inguinal hernia repair, a single-institution experience. Surg Endosc [Epub ahead of print] doi:10.1007/s00464-015-4717-5
Felix EL (2000) Extraperitoneal Hernioplasty. In: Soper NJ, Swanström LL, Eubanks WS (eds) Mastery of endoscopic and laparoscopic surgery, 1st edn. Lippincott Williams and Wilkins, Philadelphia
Felix EL, Michas CA, McKnight, RL Jr (1994) Laparoscopic herniorrhaphy. Transabdominal preperitoneal floor repair. Surg Endosc 8:103–104
Waite KE, Herman MA, Doyle PJ (2016) Comparison of robotic versus laparoscopic transabdominal preperitoneal (TAPP) inguinal hernia repair. J Robot Surg [Epub ahead of print] doi:10.1007/s11701-016-0580-1

Meshes for Inguinal Hernia Repair

14

Karl A. LeBlanc

14.1 Introduction

Synthetic mesh has now become the cornerstone of the repair of inguinal hernias. The method to repair them can be either open or laparoscopic (with or without robotic assistance). The majority of the products are a single sheet of polypropylene, polyester or expanded polytetrafluoroethylene. Currently, many of these materials are configured into a variety of shapes to facilitate the repair of the inguinal floor. Additionally, others are a combination of a permanent and an absorbable product.

Biologic mesh has been available for a number of years but has been touted for the use in ventral and incisional hernia repair. Within the last few years, a limited number of publications have described their use for inguinal hernia repair. Due to their significant cost, these products are unlikely to enjoy some of the success obtained with the other hernia repairs. These materials are generated from the dermis or small intestine of a variety of animals or cadavers.

14.2 Polypropylene Products

The flat sheets of polypropylene account for the great majority of choices for the repair of inguinal hernias (Table 14.1). Many of them can be used with either the open or laparoscopic techniques.

Basic–M is a standard-weight PPM that has a rectangular shape. This material is also configured into an "inguinal" shape and a round shape as the P3 Basic and TP bidimensional plug, respectively. There are lighter-weight versions of these materials that are called Bulev, P3 Evolution, and TP dimensional plug B. Blue

K.A. LeBlanc (✉)
Surgeons Group of Baton Rouge, Our Lady of the Lake Physician Group
Baton Rouge, Louisiana, USA
e-mail: docmba2@yahoo.com

G. Campanelli (Ed), *Inguinal Hernia Surgery,*
Updates in Surgery
DOI: 10.1007/978-88-470-3947-6_14, © Springer-Verlag Italia 2017

Table 14.1 Flat sheets of polypropylene mesh

Basic–M, *Di.pro Medical Devices, Turin, Italy*

P3 Basic, *Di.pro Medical Devices, Turin, Italy*

TP bidimensional plug, *Di.pro Medical Devices, Turin, Italy*

Bulev, *Di.pro Medical Devices, Turin, Italy*

Bulev B, *Di.pro Medical Devices, Turin, Italy*

P3 Evolution, *Di.pro Medical Devices, Turin, Italy*

P3 Evolution B, *Di.pro Medical Devices, Turin, Italy*

Bard Mesh, *Davol, Providence, RI, USA*

Bard Soft Mesh, *Davol, Providence, RI, USA*

4 D Mesh, *Cousin Biotech, Wervicq-Sud, France*

Dynamesh PP, *FEG Textiltechnik mbH, Aachen, Germany*

Dynamesh PP Light, *FEG Textiltechnik mbH, Aachen, Germany*

Hertra 1, 2, 2A, *HerniaMesh S.r.l., Turin, Italy*

Hertra 6, 6A, 7, *HerniaMesh S.r.l., Turin, Italy*

Hertra 9, 9A, *HerniaMesh S.r.l., Turin, Italy*

Hybridmesh, *HerniaMesh S.r.l., Turin, Italy*

Optilene Mesh, *B. Braun Melsungen AG, Melsungen, Germany*

Optilene Mesh LP, *B. Braun Melsungen AG, Melsungen, Germany*

Optilene Mesh Elastic, *B. Braun Melsungen AG, Melsungen, Germany*

Oval Preshaped mesh, *HerniaMesh S.r.l., Turin, Italy*

Premilene Mesh, *B. Braun Melsungen AG, Melsungen, Germany*

Premium, *Cousin Biotech, Wervicq-Sud, France*

Prolene, *Ethicon Inc., Somerville, NJ, USA*

Prolene Soft Mesh, *Ethicon Inc., Somerville, NJ, USA*

Repol Angimesh 0, 1, 8, 9, *Angiologica, S. Martino Sicc., Italy*

Surgimesh WN, *BG Medical, Barrington, IL, USA*

Surgipro, *Medtronic, Mineapolis, MN, USA*

T5 prosthesis, *HerniaMesh S.r.l., Turin, Italy*

TiMesh, *pfm medical ag, Cologne, Germany*

Tilene Blue, *pfm medical ag, Cologne, Germany*

Ultrapro, *Ethicon Inc., Somerville, NJ, USA*

strips have been added to the first two products to aid in positioning and are named Bulev B and P3 Evolution B, respectively.

Bard Mesh is a heavy-weight material and Bard Soft Mesh is a lighter weight version. Both are available as a flat sheet and a preshaped version. The 4D mesh materials are partially absorbable and come in preshapes as well. Cousin Biotech also manufactures light-weight meshes that are also preshaped as Premium. Dynamesh provides two different weights and weaves of the PPM.

A variety of Hertra meshes exist, as can be seen from the table. They differ in either thickness, stiffness and/or weave. The Hertra 1, 2, and 2A are designed to be sutureless when used with the Trabucco technique. The Hertra 6, 6A, 7 materials are light and ultralight preshaped meshes that can also be used with the sutureless technique. In addition, the Hertra 9 and 9A can also be sutureless. The Oval Preshaped mesh is designed for preperitoneal repair like the Kugel technique. The T5 prosthesis is designed also to be placed into the preperitoneal position with an additional onlay of the other meshes. Hybridmesh is a newer product that is partially absorbable and may be square, rectangular or preshaped.

The Optilene and Premilene meshes are similar to the other materials in that there are different weights of the products, which have an influence in the handling characteristics of the meshes. Prolene and Prolene Soft Mesh are also comparable materials that differ in weight and weave. The Prolene is available in preshaped, square or rectangular shapes but Prolene Soft Mesh is not preshaped. Repol Angimesh materials differ in the weight and weave of the products. They are called Repol Angimesh 0 or 1 or 8 or 9. They have a similar appearance to that of the other flat sheet meshes of polypropylene.

Surgimesh WN represents a non-woven microfiber polypropylene material that is available for non-visceral contact. It is available in several configurations. It is available as a preshaped device for Lichtenstein repair or a tear drop and "wrap around flap" for laparoscopic repair. Surgipro is one of the few prolypropylene materials available from Medtronic. It is available in multifilament, monofilament and an open weave configuration for inguinal hernia repair.

Timesh is a rather unique material that has titanized polypropylene as it base material. This can be used in the intraperitoneal position or elsewhere. Tilene Blue is the material that has blue lines to assist in the alignment of the mesh. Ultrapro mesh is a combination product that is of polypropylene but also has equal parts of absorbable poliglecaprone-25.

14.3 Polyester Materials

A greater number of these materials are available now than in the past. The most recent addition is that of the Parietex ProGrip meshes (Medtronic). These all possess an additional component of polylactic acid designed to act as a "grip" to fixate the mesh to the structure onto which it is inserted. It is available in flat sheets, a preformed product and a laparoscopic version.

Angimesh R2-1 and R2-9 are polyester materials available in flat sheets of two differing thicknesses.

14.4 Fluorinated Materials

One company manufactures materials made out of polyvinylidene fluoride (PVDF). The open mesh is called Dynamesh – Lichtenstein. Two laparoscopic versions exist, the Dynamesh Endolap and Dynamesh Endolap 3D. The more familiar expanded polytetraflurorethylene (ePTFE) products are manufactured by WL Gore & Associates (Elkhart, DE, USA). These materials are provided as the MycroMesh and MycroMesh Plus (which contains silver and chlorhexidine). The Plus product looks identical to the non-Plus product except that the silver imparts a brown color. The oldest product is that of the Soft Tissue Patch. Another configuration of the PTFE structure is condensed. This is the cPTFE material available as the Omyra mesh by B. Braun.

14.5 Plug Devices

A large number of devices have been configured roughly into the shape of a cone. There are significant differences when these are compared in terms of the selection of the base material, the exact configuration and the weight of the mesh itself (Table 14.2).

The 4D Dome product is a unique shape that has an onlay of PPM over the inguinal canal. The Easy Plug-Patch system has two different configurations of the overlap portion and is also made of the Surgimesh WN material noted above. The older plug is manufactured by Bard and comes as a heavy-weight material, Perfix Plug, but also as a lighter-weight version, Perfix Light Plug. The polyester

Table 14.2 Plug devices

4D Dome, *Cousin Biotech, Wervicq-Sud, France*
Easy Plug-Patch System, *BG Medical, Barrington, IL, USA*
Parietex Plug and Patch System, *Medtronic, Mineapolis, MN, USA*
Perfix plug, *Davol, Providence, RI*
Perfix Light plug, *Davol, Providence, RI*
Premilene Mesh Plug, *B. Braun Melsungen AG, Melsungen, Germany*
T1 plug, *HerniaMesh S.r.l., Turin, Italy*
T2 plug, *HerniaMesh S.r.l., Turin, Italy*
T3 plug, *HerniaMesh S.r.l., Turin, Italy*
T4 plug, *HerniaMesh S.r.l., Turin, Italy*
TEC–T, *Di.pro Medical Devices, Turin, Italy*
TEC–TB, *Di.pro Medical Devices, Turin, Italy*
Tilene plug and patch, *pfm medical ag, Cologne, Germany*
Ultrapro plug, *Ethicon Inc., Somerville, NJ, USA*

material Parietex has also been made into a plug with the PLA grips and is supplied with an onlay without the grips. The Premilene plug has fewer "petals" than some of the other plugs but maintains the same concept with the overlap of PPM.

Herniamesh supplies a variety of plugs, as listed in Table 14.2. The T1 plug is designed to be formed into a "dart" and inserted into the defect. The T2 is made for open repairs also and possesses a small overlay portion. The T3 has a larger overlay portion that can be modified to the floor of the inguinal canal. The T4 plug is positioned in the preperitoneal space and will also be performed with an overlay of one of the Hertra meshes discussed above.

Di.pro Medical Devices has configured the heavier-weight material of their Basic product into a three-dimensional shape that is a plug (TEC) or a plug with a flat sheet attached (TEC B). The Tilene plug-and-patch device is made from the same titanized polypropylene as the flat meshes noted above. The Ultrapro plug is of the same material as the Ultrapro above and has a different design from the other products but is also supplied with and onlay patch.

14.6 Preformed Materials

A variety of materials are made into specific shapes that can be used in either open or laparoscopic repair. The design differs depending on the application for which it is intended. The most common devices for open repair are listed in Table 14.3. These are all made of polypropylene.

The Kugel patch is an older material that is made of two pieces of mesh and is placed in the extraperitoneal position. The MK Patch also has two layers of mesh but also straps to aid in positioning and fixation. The Onflex product is designed for the open extraperitoneal method of mesh placement. It is available with or without the attached positioning straps as the Modified Onflex Mesh.

Table 14.3 Preformed materials

Kugel Patch, *Davol Inc., Warwick, RI, USA*
MK Patch, *Davol Inc., Warwick, RI, USA*
Onflex, *Davol Inc., Warwick, RI, USA*
Modified Onflex Mesh, *Davol Inc., Warwick, RI, USA*
ProFlor, *Insightra Medical Inc., Irvine, CA, USA*
Prolene Hernia System, *Ethicon Inc., Somerville, NJ, USA*
Prolene 3D Patch, *Ethicon Inc., Somerville, NJ, USA*
3D Max, Davol, Inc., Warwick, RI, USA
3D Max Light, Davol Inc., Warwick, RI, USA
Visilex, Davol Inc., Warwick, RI, USA
Ultrapro Hernia System, *Ethicon Inc., Somerville, NJ, USA*

The Prolene Hernia System and the Ultrapro Hernia System are basically the same design but the latter product is lighter weight and contains the absorbable component of poliglecaprone-25. The Prolene 3D Patch is a similar but different product that contains the overlay portion of PP but also has an "configurable plug" portion that is opened with the pull of a suture into the inguinal opening. A new product has been developed that is designed to diminish the incidence of chronic postoperative pain. These products have a 3D structure with an underlay which attempts to eliminate the use of any fixation to the anterior inguinal floor. The ProFlor products are available in differing sizes of 25 mm or 40 mm with and without a large underlay.

Several other materials that have already been discussed above can be used in either the open or laparoscopic method to repair these hernias. A few of them are specific to the latter technique. The 3D Max and 3D Max Light are made to conform to the internal shape of the inguinal floor and are made to cover the entire myopectineal orifice. The Visilex, on the other hand, is a flat sheet of PPM that has a thicker linear portion that aids in positioning of the product during this repair.

14.7   Biologic Materials

The use of biologic products in the repair of inguinal hernias has never really found a significant amount of usage. This might be due to the significant additional cost associated with the use of these materials. These meshes are made from a variety of animal or cadaveric sources. The long-term benefits of this usage are still undergoing research but the surgeon should be familiar with them. It might benefit the patient to use these products in the case of infection. However, there is no short- or long-term data to support this claim at this time.

Current available cadaveric dermal material sheets include AlloMax by Davol and Flex HD by Ethicon. Bovine materials include the SurgiMend from fetal bovine dermis by TEI Biosciences (Waltham, MA, USA). Tutopatch, the fenestrated Tutomesh (Alachua, FL, USA), and Veritas (Baxter, Deerfield, IL, USA) are from bovine pericardium.

Porcine products have a wider range of configurations but are most often indicated for complex abdominal wall reconstruction rather than inguinal hernia repair. The common mesh that is available for inguinal hernia repair are flat non-fenestrated sheets of the multilayer Biodesign tissue graft, which is made of small intestinal submucosa by Cook (Bloomington, IL, USA). It is a multilayer material and differs from all of the other biologic materials listed.

14.8   Conclusions

The use of any material to repair the inguinal floor must be chosen carefully. The surgeon should be familiar with most of these materials to perform the most effective operation for the repair of the hernia in that specific patient. A thorough knowledge of the extensive variety of mesh products will enable the operator to align the materials and the patient for optimal outcome.

Suggested Readings

LeBlanc KA (2013) Prostheses and products for hernioplasty, In: Kingsnorth AN, LeBlanc KA (eds) Management of abdominal wall hernias, 4th edn. Springer, New York, pp 103-150

Inguinal Hernia Recurrence

15

Ivy N. Haskins and Michael J. Rosen

15.1 Introduction

Inguinal hernia repair is one of the most commonly performed general surgery procedures [1, 2]. Despite its prevalence, there is no consensus regarding the optimal approach to inguinal hernia repair [2]. With an estimated recurrence rate of 0.2% to 17%, there is no doubt that recurrent inguinal hernias have a significant impact on the global healthcare system and that a durable, primary repair is ideal [3, 4]. A thorough preoperative patient evaluation, inspection of all potential locations of a groin hernia, and meticulous surgical technique all contribute to primary repair success. Nevertheless, recurrent hernias do occur and a general knowledge of the causes for a failed primary repair and surgical approach to recurrent hernias is essential. In this chapter, we will discuss the risk factors associated with inguinal hernia recurrence and the operative approach to recurrent inguinal hernia repair.

15.2 Risk Factors for Inguinal Hernia Recurrence

There are several patient and operative characteristics that increase the risk of inguinal hernia recurrence. Patient factors include malnutrition, immunosuppression, obesity, diabetes mellitus, and smoking, all of which negatively impact the wound healing process [5]. Significant time should be spent during the preoperative evaluation at minimizing or resolving these patient factors. One method that has been successful in improving preoperative optimization at our institution is engaging patients in addressing their high-risk factors. Previous studies have

I.N. Haskins (✉)
Cleveland Clinic Comprehensive Hernia Center, Department of General Surgery,
The Cleveland Clinic
Cleveland, Ohio, USA
e-mail: haskini@ccf.org

G. Campanelli (Ed), *Inguinal Hernia Surgery,*
Updates in Surgery
DOI: 10.1007/978-88-470-3947-6_15, © Springer-Verlag Italia 2017

shown that inguinal hernia recurrence is the most important long-term outcome and measure of success from a patient's perspective [6, 7]. Therefore, instilling a sense of self-responsibility in patients to their surgical outcome often leads to increased motivation to achieve preoperative goals.

Technical errors also increase the risk of inguinal hernia recurrence. Large inguinal hernias, undue tension which leads to tissue ischemia, incomplete dissection of the hernia sac, inadequate mesh size, and wound infection all increase the risk of inguinal hernia recurrence [4, 5, 8–10]. Larger groin hernias stretch and attenuate the surrounding fascial planes to a greater extent than smaller groin hernias. This leads to the incorporation of weaker tissue during repair of larger hernias as compared to smaller groin hernias [10]. As with other hernia repairs, mesh utilization has led to a more durable inguinal hernia repair, which is likely due to a reduction of medial recurrences at the pubic tubercle [4, 9]. However, incomplete coverage of the pubic tubercle or at the internal inguinal ring by prosthetic material can lead to recurrences at these sites. Recurrence at the internal ring can also be caused by improper ligation of the hernia sac [8]. General surgeons must be conscious of these risk factors during inguinal hernia repair operations in order to maximize the potential for successful primary repair.

15.3   When to Repair Recurrent Inguinal Hernias

Despite the fact that a majority of first-time and recurrent groin hernias are as-ymptomatic at presentation, the long-term teaching has been to repair these her-nias due to the perceived risk of associated bowel obstruction and/or strangulation [11, 12]. Further studies are needed to determine the ideal approach to asymptom-atic recurrent groin hernias. Nevertheless, we do recommend surgical repair of all symptomatic recurrent inguinal hernias to prevent worsening of patient symptoms and to avoid the associated risk of emergency surgery should these hernias prog-ress to bowel involvement.

15.4   Surgical Approach to Recurrent Inguinal Hernias

The European Hernia Society's (EHS) recommendation for repair of recurrent inguinal hernias is to "modify technique in relation to previous technique" [1]. Although this may seem oversimplified, approaching a recurrent inguinal hernia in a different surgical plane than the original operation leads to the best chance of repair success. The reason for this is twofold. First, surgery in a previously operated field is distorted with scar tissue. Scar tissue complicates the dissection in the inguinal canal and increases the risk for adverse outcomes such as testicular ischemia in a male patient or missing the recurrent hernia sac [3]. Second, the tissue in a healed wound is always weaker than virgin tissue. This increases the risk for recurrence with each subsequent inguinal hernia repair [3]. Therefore, review of prior operative reports requires scrutiny in an effort to avoid previous operative fields during recurrent inguinal hernia repair whenever possible.

In concert with the EHS, our recommendation for approaching recurrent inguinal hernias can be broadly categorized based on the prior failed surgical approach. Patients with a prior anterior repair (i.e., tissue repair or Lichtenstein repair) should have a posterior approach for repair of their inguinal hernia recurrence. Similarly, patients with a failed posterior approach (i.e., laparoscopic repair or Kugel repair) require an anterior repair for inguinal hernia recurrence. Finally, patients who underwent initial inguinal hernia repair in a bilaminar fashion with mesh in both the anterior and posterior compartments (i.e., Prolene Hernia System repair or plug-and-patch repair) should undergo repair of their inguinal hernia recurrence with an approach that the operating surgeon has most experience with.

15.4.1 Anterior Approach to Recurrent Inguinal Hernia Repair for Prior Failed Posterior Repairs

The anterior approach to recurrent inguinal hernia repair should be used in patients with previous posterior repairs such as laparoscopic or Kugel type repairs. The procedure of choice in these cases is a Lichtenstein repair with mesh utilization. The Lichtenstein repair is the ideal anterior approach to recurrent inguinal hernia repair after a prior posterior repair. This is because it utilizes a completely different operative field and allows for the utilization of mesh, two factors proven to decrease the risk of inguinal hernia recurrence [3, 4, 6]. For further details on the Lichtenstein repair, please refer to Chapter 1.

15.4.2 Laparoscopic Approach to Recurrent Inguinal Hernia Repair after Failed Anterior Repair

The laparoscopic approach to inguinal hernia recurrences should be used following open anterior inguinal hernia repairs. The laparoscopic approach to inguinal hernia repair includes both the transabdominal preperitoneal (TAPP) repair and the total extraperitoneal (TEP) repair. The decision to proceed with a TAPP versus a TEP repair for repair of a recurrent inguinal hernia is based largely on surgeon preference. Further details on TAPP and TEP repairs are provided in other chapters of this book.

The laparoscopic approach to recurrent inguinal hernia repair offers several advantages over the open approach to recurrent inguinal hernia repair which will be discussed. However, it should also be mentioned that a missed cord lipoma is a pitfall of the laparoscopic approach to inguinal hernia repair [13]. Therefore, should patients not have an identifiable groin hernia during laparoscopic exploration, further investigation of the preperitoneal structures should follow to rule out a missed lipoma.

The benefits of a laparoscope approach to recurrent inguinal hernia repair are numerous. Similar to the anterior approach following posterior failure, the laparoscopic approach also allows for an operation through a virgin, unscarred field following anterior inguinal hernia repair failure [3]. Furthermore, the laparoscopic platform allows for visualization of all potential hernia sites, including the femoral and obturator canals. In a study published from the Swedish Hernia Registry, 42% of women with inguinal hernia recurrence actually had a femoral hernia at the time of reoperation [14]. In addition, several other case series have found that 9% of all inguinal hernia recurrences are actually femoral hernias [3]. This underscores the fact that femoral hernias are often overlooked during open inguinal hernia repair due to lack of visualization of the femoral canal. Moreover, the laparoscopic approach to inguinal hernia recurrence may provide for a more durable repair. A previous long-term study by Bisgaard et al. found that the rate of re-recurrence following laparoscopic repair of recurrent inguinal hernia was significantly lower than the rate of re-recurrence following an anterior approach [15]. Finally, the laparoscopic approach offers the other proposed benefits to laparoscopic surgery, including decreased postoperative pain and earlier return to normal activity [3, 16, 17].

15.4.3 Approach to Inguinal Hernia Repair after Failed Anterior and Posterior Repairs

Re-recurrent inguinal hernia poses a clinical challenge to the surgeon. With each subsequent inguinal hernia repair, weaker fascia and tissue is incorporated into the repair and the risk of cord injury and testicular ischemia increases [10]. These are real risks that must be discussed with the patient during the informed consent process prior to proceeding with any surgical intervention.

Previous studies have shown that the risk of re-recurrence after laparoscopic inguinal hernia repair is significantly less than the risk of re-recurrence following Lichtenstein inguinal hernia repair [15, 18, 19]. Nevertheless, in high-risk procedures such as re-recurrent inguinal hernia repair, it is most important to be able to perform an operation that addresses the hernia recurrence while keeping the patient safe. Therefore, it is our recommendation that re-recurrent inguinal hernia repair operations be performed with the approach that is most comfortable to the surgeon. In other words, surgeons more comfortable with an anterior approach should perform a Lichtenstein repair while surgeons who are better versed at the laparoscopic approach should perform either a TAPP or a TEP. Alternatively, a Rives-Stoppa approach to re-recurrent inguinal hernia repair can be utilized. All re-recurrent inguinal hernia repairs are technically challenging and should utilize mesh for reinforcement of the weaker tissue incorporated into the repair due to operation in a previously scarred operative field.

15.5 Special Attention to the Femoral Canal

Indirect inguinal hernias remain the most common hernia in both men and women. Nevertheless, the risk of non-inguinal hernias, specifically femoral hernias, is significantly higher in women [3, 20, 21]. Furthermore, the incidence of femoral hernia repair during presumed inguinal hernia recurrence surgery is significantly higher than at primary groin hernia repair [14, 21]. Although femoral hernias are typically associated with elderly women, femoral hernias following inguinal hernia repair often occur in both middle-aged men and women [21]. The proposed pathogenesis for the increased incidence of femoral hernia following groin hernia surgery is thought to be related to either overlooking a femoral hernia present at the time of the original surgery or the spontaneous development of a femoral hernia postoperatively due to widening of the femoral canal during inguinal hernia repair [20, 21]. As femoral hernias are associated with an increased risk of emergency surgery, bowel strangulation, and postoperative morbidity and mortality, we recommend the routine exploration of the femoral canal during both primary and recurrent inguinal hernia repair operations [21, 22].

15.6 Conclusions

Inguinal hernia recurrence remains a common pathology encountered by the general surgeon. Preoperative evaluation and planning must take into consideration modifiable patient risk factors for hernia recurrence and prior surgical approaches to hernia repair. As recommended by the EHS, approach to recurrent groin hernia repair should be different than the original inguinal hernia repair whenever possible. In addition, special attention should be directed to evaluation of the femoral canal due to the increased risk of femoral hernia diagnosis during presumed recurrent inguinal hernia repair.

References

1. Kulacoglu H (2011) Current options in inguinal hernia repair in adult patients. Hippokratia 15:223–231
2. Fegade S (2008) Laparoscopic versus open repair of inguinal hernia. World J Lap Surg 1:41–48
3. Itani KMF, Fitzgibbons R, Awad SS et al (2009) Management of recurrent inguinal hernias. J Am Coll Surg 209:653–658
4. Campanelli G, Pettinari D, Cavallia M et al (2006) Inguinal hernia recurrence: classification and approach. J Minim Access Surg 2:147–150
5. Wagner JP, Brunicardi F, Amid PZ et al (2014) Inguinal hernias. In: Brunicardi F, Andersen DK, Billiar TR et al (eds) Schwartz's Principles of Surgery, 10th edn. Springer, New York
6. Haapaniemi S, Gunnarsson U, Nordin P et al (2001) Reoperation after recurrent groin hernia repair. Ann Surg 234:122–126

7. Lawrence K, McWhinnie D, Goodwin A et al (1995) Randomised controlled trial of laparoscopic versus open repair of inguinal hernia: early results. BMJ 311:981–985
8. Gilbert AI, Graham MF, Voigt WJ (2000) Inguinal hernia: anatomy and management. Medscape http://www.medscape.org/viewarticle/420354_1
9. Nillson E, Happaniemi S, Gruber G et al (1998) Methods of repair and risk for reoperation in Swedish hernia surgery from 1992 to 1996. Br J Surg 85:1686–1691
10. Javid PJ, Greenberg JA, Brooks DC et al (2013) Hernias. In: Zinner MJ, Ashley SW (eds) Maingot's Abdominal Operations, 12th edn. McGraw-Hill, New York
11. Thompson JS, Gibbs JO, Reda DJ et al (2008) Does delaying repair of an asymptomatic hernia have a penalty? Am J Surg 195:89–93
12. O'Dwyer PJ, Norrie J, Alani A et al (2006) Observation or operation for patients with an asymptomatic inguinal hernia: a randomized clinical trial. Ann Surg 244:161–173
13. Gersin KS, Heniford BT, Garcia-Ruiz A et al (1999) Missed lipoma of the spermatic cord. A pitfall of transabdominal preperitoneal laparoscopic hernia repair. Surg Endosc 13:585–587
14. Kock A, Edwards A, Haapaniemi S et al (2005) Prospective evaluation of 6895 groin hernia in women. Br J Surg 92:1553–1558
15. Bisgaard T, Bay-Nielsen M, Kehlet H (2008) Re-recurrence after operation for recurrent inguinal hernia. A nationwide 8-year follow-up study on the role of the type of repair. Ann Surg 247:707–711
16. McNally M, Byrd KA, Duncan JE et al (2009) Laparoscopic versus open inguinal hernia repair: expeditionary medical facility Kuwait experience. Military Medicine 174(12): 1320–1323
17. Karthikesalingman A, Markar SR, Holt PJ et al (2010) Meta-analysis of randomized controlled trials comparing laparoscopic with open mesh repair of recurrent inguinal hernias. Br J Surg 97:4–11
18. Bisgaard T, Bay-Nielsen M, Kehlet H (2003) Recurrence rate after laparoscopic repair of recurrent inguinal hernias: Have we improved? Surg Endosc 17:1781–1783
19. Haapaniemi S, Gunnarsson U, Nordin P et al (2001) Reoperation after recurrent groin hernia repair. Ann Surg 234:122–126
20. Henriksen NA, Thorup J, Jorgensen LN (2012) Unsuspected femoral hernia in patients with a preoperative diagnosis of recurrent inguinal hernia. Hernia 16:381–385
21. Mikkelsen T, Bay-Nielsen M, Kehlet H (2002) Risk of femoral hernia after inguinal herniorrhaphy. Br J Surg 89:486–488
22. Kjaergaard J, Bay Nielsen M, Kehlet H (2010) Mortality following emergency groin hernia surgery in Denmark. Hernia 14: 351–355

Chronic Pain after Inguinal Hernia Repair

16

Giampiero Campanelli, Piero Giovanni Bruni, Andrea Morlacchi, and Marta Cavalli

16.1 Definition and Clinical Assessment

Chronic pain is a significant long-term complication that can occur after inguinal hernia repair and can compromise the patient's quality of life. Although this complication is increasingly recognized, much controversy still exists in the literature regarding its incidence, terminology, pathogenesis and treatment strategies.

In an attempt to unify the terminology, the International guidelines for prevention and management of postoperative chronic pain following inguinal hernia surgery [1], in agreement also with the IASP (International Association for the Study of Pain) definition, proposed the following definition: a pain arising as a direct consequence of a nerve lesion or a disease affecting the somatosensory system, in patients who did not have groin pain before their original hernia operation, or, if they did, the postoperative pain differs from the preoperative pain.

The pain complex syndrome of postherniorrhaphy inguinodynia includes pain (neuralgia), burning sensation (paresthesia), hypoesthesia, hyperesthesia, with radiation of the pain to the skin of the corresponding hemiscrotum, labium majus, and Scarpa's triangle. The symptoms are frequently triggered or at least aggravated by walking, stooping, or hyperextension of the hip and can be decreased by recumbency and flexion of the thigh, suggesting that traction of the involved nerve plays a major role in the postherniorrhaphy pain syndrome. The neuropathic pain complex can also be reproduced by tapping the skin medial to the anterosuperior spine of the iliac bone or over an area of localized tenderness (Tinel's test) [2].

G. Campanelli (✉)
General and Day Surgery Unit, Center of Research and High Specialization for the Pathologies of Abdominal Wall and Surgical Treatment and Repair of Abdominal Hernia, Istituto Clinico Sant'Ambrogio
Milan, Italy
e-mail: giampiero.campanelli@grupposandonato.it

G. Campanelli (Ed), *Inguinal Hernia Surgery,*
Updates in Surgery
DOI: 10.1007/978-88-470-3947-6_16, © Springer-Verlag Italia 2017

The examination of a patient with postoperative chronic pain should always include neurophysiological assessment, preoperative characteristics (nociceptive function, pain genes, psychosocial factors, pain in other parts of the body) and the administration of a validated inguinal hernia repair specific questionnaire [1, 3, 4].

16.2 Etiology

Etiology of this pain complex syndrome includes non-neuropathic and neuropathic causes (and not infrequently a combination of both). Non-neuropathic causes include mechanical pressure of rolled-up or wadded mesh and folded prosthetic material – the so-called "meshoma" [5] – on the adjacent tissue including the vas deferens and nerves, periosteal reaction (due to a suture or staple in the pubic tubercle), or scar tissue formation. Neuropathic pain can be caused by (a) compression of one or more nerves by "perineural fibrosis", suture material, staples and tacks, prosthetic material or (b) actual nerve injury caused by partial or complete transection of nerves due to accidental cutting or excessive traction of the nerves [2].

16.3 Incidence

Regarding the incidence of chronic pain, the literature data are fairly heterogeneous: this variance (0.7–43.3%) is due to differing definitions of chronic pain, different times of assessment and different methods of measurement [1]. In the literature, the rate of debilitating pain affecting normal daily activities or work is reported to be 0.5–6% [6]. There is evidence from two randomized controlled trials that chronic pain diminishes over time [7, 8].

16.4 Risk Factors and Causes

Some risk factors for persisting postoperative pain have been identified: increased preoperative Activity Assessment Scale (AAS) score, preoperative pain to tonic heat stimulation [9], early (evaluated at one week [10] and one month [9] after surgery) postoperative pain, nerve damage (assessed as sensory dysfunction in the groin at 6 months) [9], open surgery [10] and younger age [3, 11].

16.5 Prevention of Postoperative Chronic Pain

Since surgeons cannot modify patients' risk factors for chronic pain, their attention focuses on preoperative patients selection and intraoperative features that can influence nerve damage and early postoperative pain, such as choice of the approach, identification of the nerves, choice of the mesh and its fixation.

16.5.1 Selection of patients

Patients with unusual preoperative inguinal pain in an imperceptible hernia must be evaluated with attention and often a proper physical examination and clinical history investigation reveal a different cause for their pain: back disease, hip pathologies, pubic bone or tendon injuries, etc.

Among all pathologies that can cause inguinodynia, the so-called pubic inguinal pain syndrome (PIPS) [12] or sportsman hernia is often wrongly labeled inguinal hernia and treat like it were. We want strongly underline that PIPS is a situation that can occur not only in sportsman, but also even in population with normal physical activity and that it absolutely not a real hernia. This has to be deeply kept in mind when we deal with a case of post-operative chronic pain: indeed this could be the results of a misdiagnosis and an uncorrected treatment.

So for all these reasons, it is evident that surgery should not limit the treatment to the posterior wall but also includes release of the three nerves of the region and partial calibrated tenotomy of abdominal rectus and adductor longus, otherwise preoperative pain relief cannot be completely achieved [13].

16.5.2 Choice of Technique and Approach

Different open mesh repairs (Prolene Hernia System, mesh and plug repair and Lichtenstein) have been compared and no clinically relevant differences in chronic pain have been shown on long-term outcome analysis (follow-up range, 6.9–9.2 years).

In order to decrease extensive dissection in the inguinal canal, limit manipulation of the inguinal nerves [14] and minimize interaction between the foreign material of the mesh and the spermatic cord and nerves, placement of the mesh in the preperitoneal space is an option to be considered [15]. Preperitoneal placement of the mesh can be achieved by a laparoscopic approach or by an open anterior or open posterior approach.

In a meta-analysis of all randomized controlled trials (RCTs) comparing open inguinal hernia repair and laparoscopic inguinal hernia repair for primary unilateral inguinal hernia there was a significantly reduced risk of chronic groin pain in those undergoing laparoscopic repair; on subgroup analysis, however, when the transabdominal preperitoneal (TAPP) approach was compared with the open approach, there continued to be a reduced risk of chronic groin pain, but when the totally extraperitoneal (TEP) approach was compared with the open approach, the reduced risk in chronic groin pain was not significant [16].

Willaert et al. [15] recently carried out a Cochrane review to compare the efficacy of elective open preperitoneal mesh repair (Read-Rives technique [17], transinguinal preperitoneal (TIPP [15] and Kugel patch [14]) with the Lichtenstein technique. The TIPP and Kugel patch techniques reported less chronic pain; however, slightly more chronic pain was reported after the Read-Rives technique.

16.5.3 Identification and Respect of All Three Nerves

Several patterns of nerve injury during elective inguinal hernia repair have been described, including inadvertent suture entrapment, partial division, crushing, diathermy burn, or scar encroachment [18].

Identification and routine excision or division of selected inguinal nerves during inguinal hernia repair has been proposed as a method for avoiding postoperative neuralgia [19].

Overall, even though the systematic review and meta-analysis by Hsu et al. [16] indicated that preserving the ilioinguinal nerve during open mesh repair of an inguinal hernia was associated with decreased incidence of sensory loss at 6 and 12 months postoperatively, compared with the nerve division technique, the authors found no difference between the two surgical procedures in regard to the occurrence of chronic groin pain or numbness.

For this reason, the European Hernia Society Guidelines for the treatment of inguinal hernia in adults [20] do not recommend routine prophylactic resection of the ilioinguinal nerve (Grade A).

It remains speculative whether this approach would be beneficial in a subset of patients with preoperative risk factors for chronic pain [20].

It should be noted that several studies comparing nerve preservation and prophylactic neurectomy included only the ilioinguinal nerve, forgetting that all three nerves contribute to the sensory innervation of the groin, and the majority of surgeons still fail to identify all three inguinal nerves. In fact, identification of the iliohypogastric nerve ranges between 32% [21] to 97.5% [22] of cases and that of the genital branch of the genitofemoral nerve ranges between 21.3% [22] and 36% [21] of cases.

Studies on the role of the identification of all three inguinal nerves [23, 24] concluded that identification and preservation of these nerves during open inguinal hernia repairs reduces chronic incapacitating groin pain to less than 1% and that the risk of developing inguinal chronic pain increases with the number of nerves concomitantly undetected [23].

For all these reasons, the authors strongly recommend to identify and protect all three inguinal nerves, to avoid removing the nerves from their natural bed as much as possible, and to avoid removing their covering fascia, as recommended

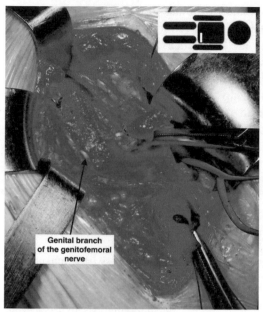

Fig. 16.1 Left inguinal region during surgery for the treatment of chronic postoperative pain: isolation of the previously placed mesh and identification of a running fixation suture along the inguinal ligament; the suture also involves the genital branch of genitofemoral nerve.

in the International guidelines [1]. Only in the event of a suspected or frankly injured nerve or its running in the way of the repair can the nerve be completely removed and its proximal cut end implanted in the muscle [1].

Care should also be taken during mesh placement to prevent the mesh from encroaching the course of the nerve (the medial edge of the mesh sometimes meets and crosses the ilioinguinal or often the iliohypogastric nerve): in this case neurectomy can be done or, preferably, a small window in the edge of the mesh can be cut so that the interaction between mesh and nerve is minimized [25, 26].

16.5.4 Choice of Mesh: Lightweight versus Heavyweight

Although the use of a synthetic mesh substantially reduces the risk of hernia recurrence [27], polypropylene meshes have been found to cause chronic inflammatory reactions that persist for years and can have potentially negative effects, including chronic pain [28].

It has been hypothesized that the extent of the foreign body reaction with its provoked scar tissue is correlated with the amount of the synthetic material used [29]. This has led to the development of so-called lightweight meshes characterized by a reduction in the polypropylene volume, an increase in the pore size, or different web structure [30, 31].

In open groin hernia surgery, several meta-analyses of RCTs have now shown that lightweight (flat) meshes do not have an advantage in the short term, but are associated with less chronic (>6 months) pain and foreign body sensation [32, 33], although the incidence of severe chronic groin pain is not decreased [34]. Importantly, this does not increase the recurrence rate (follow up range, 6–60 months), although caution is still needed in large (direct) hernias with a potential increased risk for mesh migration into the defect, especially when some specific points for mesh fixation are not taken into account [35–40]. There is not sufficient evidence for such recommendation in endoscopic groin hernia repair [41], with respect to either short- or long-term outcomes.

16.5.5   Choice of Fixation

Penetrating fixating or traumatic devices like sutures, staples and tacks cause local trauma that may result in nerve injury and chronic pain and should therefore be used with caution (Fig. 16.1).

A multicenter RCT [42] has suggested that fibrin sealant may have a beneficial effect in chronic pain. In the recent systematic review proposed by Sanders [43], twelve trials comparing n-butyl-2 cyanoacrylate (NB2C) glues to sutures, self-fixing meshes to sutures, fibrin sealant to sutures, tacks to sutures and absorbable sutures to non-absorbable sutures were included. Although there was no significant difference in recurrence or surgical site infection rates between fixation methods, there is insufficient evidence to promote fibrin sealant, self-fixing meshes or NB2C glues ahead of suture fixation.

Although several studies [44–52] have compared the type of fixation in the laparoscopic approach (none vs. atraumatic vs. resorbable or non-resorbable fixation devices), the analysis is seriously flawed by different factors such as the way chronic pain is evaluated and the many independent variables (the type of repair, the type of hernia, the type of mesh and the type, number and location of the fixation devices). Thus recommendations from the European guidelines are that, when using heavyweight meshes, traumatic mesh fixation in TEP endoscopic repair should be avoided (with the exception of some cases such as large direct hernias). Atraumatic mesh fixation in TAPP endoscopic repair can be used without increasing the recurrence rate at 1 year.

16.6   Treatment

Data in the literature are poor and inconsistent due to limited information on preoperative demographics, differences in definition and evaluation of pain degree and limited follow-up, so comparison among different strategies and their results is very difficult.

Initial acute postoperative pain treatment should be as effective as possible and standard pharmacological pain treatment (gabapentanoids, tricyclics, etc.) [53]

for neuropathic pain should be instituted earlier in patients with severe pain. The question of whether this may reduce development of chronic pain is debatable in the absence of any conclusive data [54]. The working group of the international guidelines for prevention and management of postoperative chronic pain following inguinal hernia repair decided to consider reasonable surgical treatment only after 1 year postoperatively, when the inflammatory response has decreased, and only when pain intensity curtails activity and conventional treatment has failed (level of evidence 5, grade of recommendation "D") [1].

It has been proved that analgesic patches [lidocaine patch (5%) and capsaicin (8%)] do not reduce summed pain intensity (at rest, during movement, and during pressure) [55].

Nerve infiltration with anesthetics is a minimally invasive technique for treating peripheral neuropathy after inguinal surgery [56, 57]. Varying success rates have been reported, but the relative ease of application is a main advantage [58, 59]. Several studies [60–68] reported the use of diagnostic blocks presurgery. The use of ultrasound-guided regional anesthesia has increased in the last decade and enables direct visualization of peripheral nerves, facilitating the success rate of the blocks [58]. As a result, there is no scientific evidence of any short-term or long-term analgesic efficacy of local anesthetic blocks in persistent postsurgical pain (PPP) following inguinal hernia repair. However, the potential for local anesthetic blocks in predicting surgical outcome should be considered, particularly in excision of painful neuromas [69]: e.g., if a diagnostic nerve block is ineffective in relieving pain, patients will most likely not benefit from surgical treatment.

Several different techniques of neuromodulation have been proposed. Pulsed radiofrequency (PRF) is an invasive pain treatment technique that employs electromagnetic energy deposited in or near nerve tissue [70, 71]. An insulated needle with an active tip is inserted at the vertebral level or at the peripheral level. Paresthesias are then elicited in the painful area, by electrical stimulation as an indication of adequate positioning of the needle tip. The voltage applied to the treatment needle is rapidly raised and lowered, with voltages typically alternating between 0 and 40 V with a frequency of 300–500 kHz. The temperature is held below 42°C avoiding structural damage to the nerve tissue. The moderate heating of the nerve tissue is believed to temporarily block the nerve conduction.

Conventional continuous radiofrequency (CRF) produces temperatures at the tip of the treatment needle of 45–80°C leading to irreversible thermo-coagulation of nerve structures and has proven considerably more efficacious than PRF in various chronic pain states [70]. A recent retrospective uncontrolled study reported a longer duration of pain relief in the CRF group than in the local anesthetic block group at 12-month follow-up [72].

Peripheral nerve stimulation utilizing a transperitoneal laparoscopic approach with selective implantation of quadripolar electrodes at the genitofemoral nerve (anterior surface psoas major muscle) or ilioinguinal nerve, iliohypogastric nerve and femoro-cutaneous lateral nerve (anterior surface quadratus lumborum muscle) has recently been presented with promising results [73].

Although preliminary reports with neuromodulation techniques are enthusiastic and promising, the evidence is still of low quality, and the strength of recommendation is weak to moderate [71]. The scientific rigor is generally not considered adequate and study designs should be improved in regard to control groups, randomization, blinding procedures, and adequate sampling sizes [74].

Werner [74] reported a comprehensive review of 25 studies [2, 60–66, 75–89] in the surgical management of PPP following inguinal hernia repair. Most of the studies reported an open surgical approach, few a laparoscopic approach and only three studies reported a combined approach. All studies included neurectomy and comprise selective neurectomy, triple neurectomy or extended neurectomy. Removal of the mesh, either complete or partial, was performed in 11 studies and a new mesh was placed in five studies. Consistently satisfactory results in the majority of patients were reported.

With regard to follow-up, it is important to remember that nerve transection is known be associated with delayed onset of neuropathic pain symptoms, from months to years, so extended follow-up times are suggested [74].

In spite of these shortcomings, the data on surgical management clearly demonstrate that neurectomy with or without mesh removal may provide long-lasting analgesic effects in most patients with severe PPP following inguinal hernia repair.

The authors propose a total simultaneous double approach to the inguinal region: first, by a posterior-preperitoneal approach we identify and cut all the sensitive nerves, and safely remove the plug (if any) placed during previous surgery and then, by an anterior approach through the same incision, we remove the mesh and fixation stitches placed during previous surgery. A new repair is done with an ultralight or biological mesh in the preperitoneal space fixed with glue [75].

We always perform a triple neurectomy as it is extremely difficult, if not impossible, to pinpoint the involved nerve because peripheral communication between the ilioinguinal, iliohypogastric, and genital branch of the genital femoral nerve is very common and results in an overlap of their sensory innervation. The preperitoneal approach allows us to identify the three nerves in a virgin field without scarring. Finally, we always remove the previously placed mesh because the real reason for pain (neuropathic or non-neuropathic) cannot be detected.

References

1. Alfieri S, Amid PK, Campanelli G et al (2011) International guidelines for prevention and management of post-operative chronic pain following inguinal hernia surgery. Hernia 15:239–249
2. Amid PK (2004) Causes, prevention and surgical treatment of postherniorrhaphy neuropathic inguinodynia: triple neurectomy with proximal end implantation. Hernia 8:343–349
3. Kehlet H, Jensen TS, Woolf CJ (2006) Persistent postsurgical pain: risk factors and prevention. Lancet 367:1618–1625
4. Franneby U, Gunnarsson U, Andersson M et al (2008) Validation of an inguinal pain

questionnaire for assessment of chronic pain after groin hernia repair. Br J Surg 95:488–493

5. Amid PK (2004) Radiological images of meshoma: a new phenomenon after prosthetic repair of abdominal wall hernia. Arch Surg 139:1297–1298

6. Kehlet H (2008) Chronic pain after groin hernia repair. Br J Surg 95:135–136

7. van Veen RN, Wijsmuller AR, Vrijland WW et al (2007) Randomized clinical trial of mesh versus non-mesh primary inguinal hernia repair: long-term chronic pain at 10 years. Surgery 142:695–698

8. Eklund A, Montgomery A, Bergkvist L, Rudberg C (2010) Chronic pain 5 years after randomized comparison of laparoscopic and Lichtenstein inguinal hernia repair. Br J Surg 97:600–608

9. Aasvang EK, Gmaehle E, Hansen JB et al (2010) Predictive risk factors for persistent postherniotomy pain. Anesthesiology 112:957–969

10. Singh AN, Bansal VK, Misra MC et al (2012) Testicular functions, chronic groin pain, and quality of life after laparoscopic and open mesh repair of inguinal hernia: a prospective randomized controlled trial. Surg Endosc 26:1304–1317

11. Macrae WA (2008) Chronic post-surgical pain: 10 years on. Br J Anaesth 101:77–86

12. Campanelli G (2010). Pubic inguinal pain syndrome: the so-called sports hernia. Hernia; 14(1):1-4.

13. Cavalli M, Bombini G, Campanelli G (2014). Pubic inguinal pain syndrome: the so-called sports hernia. Surg Technol Int.;24:189-94.

14. Alfieri S, Rotondi F, Di Giorgio A et al (2006) Influence of preservation versus division of ilioinguinal, iliohypogastric, and genital nerves during open mesh herniorrhaphy: prospective multicentric study of chronic pain. Ann Surg 243:553–558

15. Izard G, Gailleton R, Randrianasolo S, Houry R (1996) Treatment of inguinal hernia by McVay's technique. A propos of 1332 cases. Ann Chir 50:775–776

16. O'Reilly EA, Burke J, O'Connell PR (2012) A meta-analysis of surgical morbidity and recurrence after laparoscopic and open repair of primary unilateral inguinal hernia. Ann Surg 255:846–853

17. Campanelli G, Cavalli M, Morlacchi A, Pavoni GM (2016) Prevention of pain: optimizing the open primary inguinal hernia repair technique. In: Jacob BP, Chen DC, Ramshaw B, Twofigh S (eds) The SAGES Manual of Groin Pain. Springer International Publishing AG Switzerland

18. Nienhuijs S, Staal E, Keemers-Gels M et al (2007) Pain after open preperitoneal repair versus Lichtenstein repair: a randomized trial. World J Surg 31:1751–1757

19. Willaert W, De Bacquer D, Rogiers X et al (2012) Open preperitoneal techniques versus Lichtenstein repair for elective inguinal hernias (Review). Cochrane Database Syst Rev 7:CD008034

20. Muldoon RL, Marchant K, Johnson DD et al (2004) Lichtenstein vs anterior preperitoneal prosthetic mesh placement in open inguinal hernia repair: a prospective randomized trial. Hernia 8:98–103

21. Mui WL, Ng CS, Fung TM et al (2006) Prophylactic ilioinguinal neurectomy in open inguinal hernia repair: a double-blind randomized controlled trial. Ann Surg 244:27–33

22. Johner A, Faulds J, Wiseman M (2011) Planned ilioinguinal nerve excision for prevention of chronic pain after inguinal hernia repair: a meta-analysis. Surgery 150:534–541

23. Hsu W, Chen CS, Lee HC et al (2012) Preservation versus division of ilioinguinal nerve on open mesh repair of inguinal hernia: a meta-analysis of randomized controlled trials. World J Surg 36:2311–2319

24. Miserez M, Peeters E, Aufenacker T et al (2014) Update with level 1 studies of the European Hernia Society guidelines on the treatment of inguinal hernia in adult patients. Hernia 18:151–163

25. Wijsmuller AR, Lange JF, van Geldere D et al (2007) Surgical techniques preventing chronic pain after Lichtenstein hernia repair: state-of-the-art vs daily practice in the Netherlands. Hernia 11:147–151

26. Bischoff JM, Aasvang EK, Kehlet H, Werner MU (2012) Does nerve identification during

open inguinal herniorrhaphy reduce the risk of nerve damage and persistent pain? Hernia 16:573–577

27. Van Veen RN, Wijsmuller AR, Vrijland WW et al (2007) Long-term follow-up of a randomized clinical trial of non-mesh versus mesh repair of primary inguinal hernia. Br J Surg 94:506–510

28. Klinge U, Klosterhalfen B, Muller M, Schumpelick V (1999) Foreign body reaction to meshes used for the repair of abdominal wall hernias. Eur J Surg 165:665–673

29. Rutkow IM, Robbins AW (1993) Demographic, classificatory, and socioeconomic aspects of hernia repair in the United States. Surg Clin North Am 73:413–426

30. Greca FH, de Paula JB, Biondo-Simoes ML et al (2001) The influence of differing pore sizes on the biocompatibility of two polypropylene meshes in the repair of abdominal defects. Experimental study in dogs. Hernia 5:59–64

31. Klosterhallfen B, Klinge U, Hermanns B, Schumpelick V (2000) Pathology of traditional surgical nets for hernia repair after longterm implantation in humans. Chirurg 71:43–51

32. Sajid MS, Leaver C, Baig MK, Sains P (2012) Systematic review and meta-analysis of the use of lightweight versus heavyweight mesh in open inguinal hernia repair. Br J Surg 99:29–37

33. Uzzaman MM, Ratnasingham K, Ashraf N (2012) Meta-analysis of randomized controlled trials comparing lightweight and heavyweight mesh for Lichtenstein inguinal hernia repair. Hernia 16:505–518

34. Śmietański M, Śmietańska IA, Modrzejewski A et al (2012) Systematic review and meta-analysis on heavy and lightweight polypropylene mesh in Lichtenstein inguinal hernioplasty. Hernia 16:519–528

35. O'Dwyer PJ, Kingsnorth AN, Molloy RG et al G (2005) Randomized clinical trial assessing impact of a lightweight or heavyweight mesh on chronic pain after inguinal hernia repair. Br J Surg 92:166–170

36. Bringman S, Wollert S, Osterberg J et al (2006) Three-year results of a randomized clinical trial of lightweight or standard polypropylene mesh in Lichtenstein repair of primary inguinal hernia. Br J Surg 93:1056–1059

37. Polish Hernia Study Group, Śmietański M (2008) Randomized clinical trial comparing a polypropylene with a poliglecaprone and polypropylene composite mesh for inguinal hernioplasty. Br J Surg 95:1462–146

38. Nikkolo C, Murruste M, Vaasna T et al (2012) Three-year results of randomised clinical trial comparing lightweight mesh with heavyweight mesh for inguinal hernioplasty. Hernia 16:555–559

39. Smietański M, Bury K, Smietańska IA et al (2011) Five-year results of a randomised controlled multi-centre study comparing heavy-weight knitted versus low-weight, non-woven polypropylene implants in Lichtenstein hernioplasty. Hernia 15:495–501

40. Bury K, Smietański M (2012) Five-year results of a randomized clinical trial comparing a polypropylene mesh with a poliglecaprone and polypropylene composite mesh for inguinal hernioplasty. Hernia 16:549–553

41. Currie A, Andrew H, Tonsi A et al (2012) Lightweight versus heavyweight mesh in laparoscopic inguinal hernia repair: a meta-analysis. Surg Endosc 26:2126–2133

42. Campanelli G, Pascual M, Hoeferlin A et al (2012) Randomized, controlled, blinded trial of Tisseel/Tissucol for mesh fixation in patients undergoing Lichtenstein technique for primary inguinal hernia repair: results of the TIMELI trial. Ann Surg 255:650–657

43. Sanders DL, Waydia S (2014) A systematic review of randomised control trials assessing mesh fixation in open inguinal hernia repair. Hernia 18:165–176

44. Tam KW, Liang HH, Chai CY (2010) Outcomes of staple fixation of mesh versus nonfixation in laparoscopic total extraperitoneal inguinal repair: a meta-analysis of randomized controlled trials. World J Surg 34:3065–3074

45. Teng YJ, Pan SM, Liu YL et al (2011) A meta-analysis of randomized controlled trials of fixation versus nonfixation of mesh in laparoscopic total extraperitoneal inguinal hernia repair. Surg Endosc 25:2849–2858

46. Sajid MS, Ladwa N, Kalra L et al (2012) A meta-analysis examining the use of tacker fixation

versus no-fixation of mesh in laparoscopic inguinal hernia repair. Int J Surg 10:224–231

47.   Lau H (2005) Fibrin sealant versus mechanical stapling for mesh fixation during endoscopic extraperitoneal inguinal hernioplasty: a randomized prospective trial. Ann Surg 24:670–675

48.   Lovisetto F, Zonta S, Rota E et al (2007) Use of human fibrin glue (Tissucol) versus staples for mesh fixation in laparoscopic transabdominal preperitoneal hernioplasty: a prospective, randomized study. Ann Surg 245:222–231

49.   Olmi S, Scaini A, Erba L et al (2007) Quantification of pain in laparoscopic transabdominal preperitoneal (TAPP) inguinal hernioplasty identifies marked differences between prosthesis fixation systems. Surgery 142:40–46

50.   Boldo E, Armelles A, Perez de Lucia G et al (2008) Pain after laparoscopic bilateral hernioplasty: early results of a prospective randomized double-blind study comparing fibrin versus staples. Surg Endosc 22:1206–1209

51.   Fortelny RH, Petter-Puchner AH, May C et al (2012) The impact of atraumatic fibrin sealant vs staple mesh fixation in TAPP hernia repair on chronic pain and quality of life: results of a randomized controlled study. Surg Endosc 26:249–254

52.   Brugger L, Bloesch M, Ipaktchi R et al (2012) Objective hypoesthesia and pain after transabdominal preperitoneal hernioplasty: a prospective, randomized study comparing tissue adhesive vs spiral tack. Surg Endosc 26:1079–108

53.   Finnerup NB, Otto M, McQuay HJ et al (2005) Algorithm for neuropathic pain treatment: an evidence based proposal. Pain 118:289–305

54.   Brennan TJ, Kehlet H (2005) Preventive analgesia to reduce wound hyperalgesia and persistent postsurgical pain: not an easy path. Anesthesiology 103:681–683

55.   Bischoff JM, Petersen M, Uceyler N et al (2012) Lidocaine patch (5%) in treatment of persistent inguinal postherniorrhaphy pain: a randomized, double-blind, placebo-controlled crossover trial. Anesthesiology 119:1444–1452

56.   Carr DB (2011) Local anesthetic blockade for neuralgias: "why is the sky blue, daddy?". Anesth Analg 112:1283–1285

57.   Kissin I, Vlassakov KV, Narang S (2011) Local anesthetic blockade of peripheral nerves for treatment of neuralgias: systematic analysis. Anesth Analg 112:1487–1493

58.   Bischoff JM, Koscielniak-Nielsen ZJ, Kehlet H, Werner MU (2012) Ultrasound-guided ilioinguinal/iliohypogastric nerve blocks for persistent inguinal postherniorrhaphy pain: a randomized, double-blind, placebo-controlled, crossover trial. Anesth Analg 114:1323–1329

59.   Vlassakov KV, Narang S, Kissin I (2011) Local anesthetic blockade of peripheral nerves for treatment of neuralgias: systematic analysis. Anesth Analg 112:1487–1493

60.   Starling JR, Harms BA (1989) Diagnosis and treatment of genitofemoral and ilioinguinal neuralgia. World J Surg 13:586–591

61.   Kim DH, Murovic JA, Tiel RL, Kline DG (2005) Surgical management of 33 ilioinguinal and iliohypogastric neuralgias at Louisiana State University Health Sciences Center. Neurosurgery 56:1013–1020

62.   Rosen MJ, Novitsky YW, Cobb WS et al (2006) Combined open and laparoscopic approach to chronic pain following open inguinal hernia repair. Hernia 10:20–24

63.   Keller JE, Stefanidis D, Dolce CJ et al (2008) Combined open and laparoscopic approach to chronic pain after inguinal hernia repair. Am Surg 74:695–700

64.   Giger U, Wente MN, Büchler MW et al (2009) Endoscopic retroperitoneal neurectomy for chronic pain after groin surgery. Br J Surg 96:1076–1081

65.   Vuilleumier H, Hubner M, Demartines N (2009) Neuropathy after herniorrhaphy: indication for surgical treatment and outcome. World J Surg 33:841–845

66.   Zacest AC, Magill ST, Anderson VC, Burchiel KJ (2010) Long-term outcome following ilioinguinal neurectomy for chronic pain. J Neurosurg 112:784–789

67.   Loos MJ, Scheltinga MR, Roumen RM (2010) Tailored neurectomy for treatment of postherniorrhaphy inguinal neuralgia. Surgery 147:275–281

68.   Chen DC, Hiatt JR, Amid PK (2013) Operative management of refractory neuropathic inguinodynia by a laparoscopic retroperitoneal approach. JAMA Surg 148:962–967

69.   Stokvis A, van der Avoort DJ, van Neck JW et al (2010) Surgical management of neuroma

pain: a prospective follow up study. Pain 151:862–869

70. Chua NH, Vissers KC, Sluijter ME (2011) Pulsed radiofrequency treatment in interventional pain management: mechanisms and potential indications–a review. Acta Neurochir (Wien) 153:763–771

71. Werner MU, Bischoff JM, Rathmell JP, Kehlet H (2012) Pulsed radiofrequency in the treatment of persistent pain after inguinal herniotomy: a systematic review. Reg Anesthesiol Pain 37:340–343

72. Kastler A, Aubry S, Piccand V et al (2012) Radiofrequency neurolysis versus local nerve infiltration in 42 patients with refractory chronic inguinal neuralgia. Pain Physician 15:237–244

73. Possover M (2013) Use of the LION procedure on the sensitive branches of the lumbar plexus for the treatment of intractable postherniorrhaphy neuropathic inguinodynia. Hernia 17:333–337

74. Werner MU (2014) Management of persistent postsurgical inguinal pain. Langenbecks Arch Surg 399:559–569

75. Campanelli G, Bertocchi V, Cavalli M et al (2013) Surgical treatment of chronic pain after inguinal hernia repair. Hernia 17:347–353

76. Starling JR, Harms BA, Schroeder ME, Eichman PL (1987) Diagnosis and treatment of genitofemoral and ilioinguinal entrapment neuralgia. Surgery 102:581–586

77. Bower S, Moore BB, Weiss SM (1996) Neuralgia after inguinal hernia repair. Am Surg 62:664–667

78. Heise CP, Starling JR (1998) Mesh inguinodynia: a new clinical syndrome after inguinal herniorrhaphy? J Am Coll 187:514–518

79. Lee CH, Dellon AL (2000) Surgical management of groin pain of neural origin. J Am Coll Surg 191:137–142

80. Deysine M, Deysine GR, Reed WP Jr (2002) Groin pain in the absence of hernia: a new syndrome. Hernia 6:64–67

81. Amid PK (2002) A 1-stage surgical treatment for postherniorrhaphy neuropathic pain: triple neurectomy and proximal end implantation without mobilization of the cord. Arch Surg 137:100–104

82. Madura JA, Madura JA 2nd, Copper CM, Worth RM (2005) Inguinal neurectomy for inguinal nerve entrapment: an experience with 100 patients. Am J Surg 189:283–287

83. Amid PK, Hiatt JR (2007) New understanding of the causes and surgical treatment of postherniorrhaphy inguinodynia and orchalgia. J Am Coll Surg 205:381–385

84. Ducic I, West J, Maxted W (2008) Management of chronic postoperative groin pain. Ann Plast Surg 60:294–298

85. Aasvang EK, Kehlet H (2009) The effect of mesh removal and selective neurectomy on persistent postherniotomy pain. Ann Surg 249:327–334

86. Amid PK, Chen DC (2011) Surgical treatment of chronic groin and testicular pain after laparoscopic and open preperitoneal inguinal hernia repair. J Am Coll Surg 213:531–536

87. Koopmann MC, Yamane BH, Starling JR (2011) Long-term follow-up after meshectomy with acellular human dermis repair for postherniorraphy inguinodynia. Arch Surg 146:427–431

88. Bischoff JM, Enghuus C, Werner MU, Kehlet H (2013) Long-term follow-up after mesh removal and selective neurectomy for persistent inguinal postherniorrhaphy pain. Hernia 17:339–345

89. Valvekens E, Nijs Y, Miserez M (2015) Long-term outcome of surgical treatment of chronic postoperative groin pain: a word of caution. Hernia 19:587–594

Pubic Inguinal Pain Syndrome (PIPS): the Sportsman's Hernia

17

Aali J. Sheen, Waqar Bhatti, Max Fehily, Saurabh Jamdar, David Jones, and Doug Jones

17.1 Introduction

The concept of groin pain has been explored in many studies, with most finding the exact etiology of the so called "sportsman's groin" difficult to pinpoint [1]. This term has been "loosely" associated with a painful groin that develops in persons that undertake some degree of sporting physical activity [2]. It is well recognized though that no true hernia exists, so whether the term "hernia" should be used at all is a common theme debated in the hernia circles [3]. In Europe, the term "pubic inguinal pain syndrome" (PIPS) is preferred but across the Atlantic in the United States, "athletic pubalgia" is more commonly used and preferred [4]. Recently, a consensus meeting in Manchester concluded that "inguinal disruption" is the most logical terminology as it will accurately define a recognized physiological weakness that occurs in the inguinal canal and hence cause groin pain [3]. However, this has since been challenged with the term "inguinal-related pain" by a statement produced from a body of leading experts in a specially convened meeting in Doha [5]. Therefore, a need and challenge remains to accurately define the popularly termed "sportsman's hernia", as well as distinguish it from chronic groin pain.

The large majority of patients that present with groin pain do so by describing pain either and/or around the inguinal ligament, the perineum, the origin of the adductor tendon and the pubic symphysis (lower abdomen). The pain can be described as a persistent ache, which is exacerbated on physical activity, but also can present only on exercise with no symptoms in between or at rest. The pain is usually exacerbated with kicking, running, coughing and sneezing with

A.J. Sheen (✉)
Department of General and Hernia Surgery, Central Manchester Foundation Trust,
Manchester Royal Infirmary
Manchester, United Kingdom
e-mail: aali.sheen@cmft.nhs.uk

G. Campanelli (Ed), *Inguinal Hernia Surgery,*
Updates in Surgery
DOI: 10.1007/978-88-470-3947-6_17, © Springer-Verlag Italia 2017

these being some of the cardinal symptoms experienced [3]. It is also understood that sports which involve multidirectional change in movements with or without kicking are more likely to predispose to PIPS [4]. Football (soccer), ice & field hockey, rugby and martial arts are the kind of sports that are more likely to present with PIPS, with swimmers and cyclists less likely to do so [3, 4]. Amateur athletes tend to present at a later stage in life, due to their significantly reduced physical activity and workload, although the nature of the sporting activities is similar to the elite athletes [6].

17.1.1 Definitions

With all the definitions that have been highlighted above, it is important to critique why these definitions have been promoted. Firstly, it is generally accepted that the term "sportsman's groin" was used as this condition of a painful groin presented mainly in professional and amateur persons that undertook sports. "Athletic pubalgia" was described as a pathology which arose from the groin, where there was no true hernia and no clear-cut cause identified from the structures in the pubic region – hence the term "pubalgia" was introduced [7]. It was also understood that multiple coexisting pathologies are often present such as posterior inguinal canal weakness, conjoint or adductor tendinopathy(s), osteitis pubis and peripheral nerve entrapment syndrome [3]. "Inguinal disruption" concentrated on the fact that there are differential reasons in the groin for pain, but by a process of elimination, if the other causes such as hip impingement and adductor injuries are excluded then a weakness in the integrity of the inguinal canal was the most likely cause [3].

The Manchester statement also understood that one or more pathologies may coexist but inguinal disruption may be the predominant cause of the pain experienced. Manchester was formulated after a meeting of experts from a multidisciplinary background [3].

The Doha statement preferred the definition "inguinal-related pain" which attempted to further recognize and then re-categorize all the possible causes of groin pain with a clever subdivision using the Delphi method [4].

Inguinal-related groin pain is labeled as a defined clinical entity, which helps allude to the fact that the pain is arising possibly from the inguinal canal [4]. The methodology used for this statement was quite robust as there was an initial exercise with the expert panel being asked to make a diagnosis on three cases presented to them. A natural plethora of answers consequently led to the need for a reasonable diagnostic and descriptive terminology. "Pubic inguinal pain syndrome" is a term that has been coined and utilized mainly in Europe and arose as a result of no clear evidence but merely recognition of a condition that has a multidisciplinary etiology centred around the groin and pubic area [4, 8]. However, despite all the terminologies used, none of which allude to a true hernia being evident, there are some reports of an undetectable direct inguinal hernia as the cause [9] as well as "tears" in the external oblique aponeurosis as described by Gilmore [10].

So why does pain in the groin create so many differing definitions, which may essentially be labeling an identical pathology?

This chapter will detail the causes of groin pain and refer to the condition as PIPS to provide consistency for the reader and then discuss what investigations are deemed not only necessary but essential with a recommended guide to treatment, which may be surgical or non-surgical.

17.2 Differential Diagnosis

17.2.1 Inguinal-related Pain

Anatomy of the groin, albeit a small area, is rather complex. The inguinal ligament itself arises from the anterior superior iliac spine and inserts into the pubic tubercle, from which also arises both the rectus abdominis muscle and the adductor longus tendon. Therefore, there are a number of forces that are either "pulling" or "pushing" at the pubic bone and over time this can present with pain as illustrated in Fig. 17.1. In addition, the inguinal canal has two congenital weaknesses with the internal and external inguinal rings, both of which can be under "tension" with the eventual diminution in their respective strengths. This weakness can be recognized as a "posterior wall weakness" on dynamic

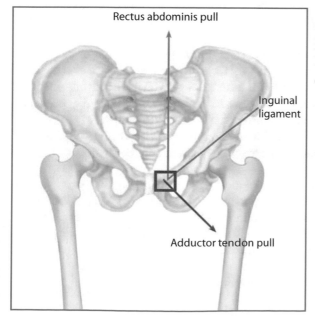

Rectus abdominis pull

Inguinal ligament

Adductor tendon pull

Fig. 17.1 Anatomical illustration depicting the inguinal ligament, adductor longus and rectus abdominis with their respective "forces" on the pubic tubercle

ultrasound imaging as described below [11]. The inguinal canal nerve anatomy may bear some relevance with a "subjective" opinion of the genital branch of the genitofemoral nerve being under "tension". Division of this nerve has therefore been advocated as a remedy, which will of course make the groin insensate and hence eliminate any pain experienced [12]. This surgical technique though has not been widely accepted or practiced and increasingly should now be tested in a trial setting.

Clinical examination therefore relies on testing all the possible differentials [13]: femoroacetabular impingement (FAI), labral tears, adductor tendinopathy, osteitis pubis and a symphyseal injury

A thorough assessment of the hip and adductor strengths is essential as well as testing a patient's balance, spinal curvature and of course groin tenderness, especially along the inguinal canal and pubic tubercle. PIPS can then be diagnosed if the three out of five clinical signs exist as per the Manchester consensus statement [3].

17.2.2 Hip-related Pain

Pathology of the hip joint is a well-recognized cause of groin pain. The most common cause in the athletic population is femoroacetabular impingement (FAI). This is a condition where there is an abnormality in the shape of either the femoral head or the shape or position of the acetabulum.

In males, the most common pathology is a prominence at the head-neck junction called a cam deformity. As the hip flexes up, this prominence impacts against the bony rim of the acetabulum and the soft cartilaginous rim (labrum) that is attached to it. Repeated flexion can cause labral tears and shear stresses at the chondrolabral junction, which in turn can lead to cartilage delamination and joint degeneration. The etiology of both pathologies is not though fully understood. The presence of a symptomatic cam deformity does seem to be more common in the athletic population [14] and probably begins to form in early adolescence. It is more commonly seen on the right hand side as that tends to be the dominant side [15]. Pincer abnormalities also start to develop in adolescence and may be associated with a gradual change in acetabular orientation as the person matures [16].

It is clear that the development of symptomatic impingement requires a combination of factors: combining an anatomical abnormality with both the type and level of activity.

Symptomatic hip impingement is most common in certain sports such as distance running, football, rugby, squash and martial arts [17,18]. All of these involve repetitive loading and unloading of the hip. It is less common in non-impact sports such as swimming and cycling as noted above. Interestingly, it is also common in sports such as gymnastics and ballet, but this may be due to impingement occurring secondary to an abnormal hip range of movement, rather than the presence of significant cam or pincer deformities [15].

Patients usually present with deep-seated antero-lateral groin pain. It tends to be in the middle or just lateral to the mid-inguinal point and exacerbated by exercise. It is not affected by coughing or raised intra-abdominal pressure, which does differentiate it from PIPS. When present for some time, it can be associated with soft-tissue pain and tendinopathy in the surrounding musculature. Patients can often present with an associated anterior clicking as the leg moves from flexion to extension and this is usually due to a psoas tendinopathy. As well as this, it is relatively common for patients to have associated pain in their lower back, sacro-iliac joint and tendinopathy in the gluteal, sartorius and adductors regions.

Clinical examination can confirm the presence of soft-tissue tenderness, and deep hip flexion, particularly with internal rotation and adduction, will often trigger the presenting pain.

Finally, because it is well recognized that it is possible to have FAI features but be asymptomatic, the use of intra-articular local anaesthetic injections (plus or minus steroids/hyaluronic acid) can be a very useful diagnostic tool in differentiating hip and inguinal pain [19].

There have been increasing numbers of published papers looking at patient outcome following hip arthroscopy for FAI. Initially, these tended to be single surgeon series with an emphasis on athletes and showed improved outcomes with good return to sport. Recently there have been a number of reviews looking at both athletic and non-athletic patients. These have shown significant improvement across both groups with regard to return to activity, as well as improvement in patient-reported outcome measures (PROMs).

17.2.3 Adductor-related Pain

On clinical evaluation, pain elicited over the inguinal ligament is more indicative of inguinal-related pain (PIPS) with more inferior pain suggestive of an adductor-related pathology [20], although it is accepted that an adductor tendinopathy can coexist with PIPS in as many as 50% of the patients [21]. As already mentioned, sports that require the strong eccentric contraction are more likely to promote a groin injury and this is especially true for adductor injuries [22]. The main action of the adductor muscle group is to adduct the thigh in the open kinetic chain and stabilize the lower extremity to any changes in all planes of motion in the closed kinetic chain. The adductor longus is the most likely muscle in this group to be injured [23]. It may be that the adductor longus's lack of mechanical advantage (due to its anatomical origin and insertion) possibly renders it more susceptible to a strain. As discussed later, the need to strengthen and improve the stability of the adductor muscle group becomes essential in reducing the time an athlete spends away from their sport as well avoiding the need for any operative intervention [24].

17.3   Imaging Investigations

The diagnosis and correct management of the sports-related groin pain, PIPS, is extremely challenging for the practising clinician who is reliant on both clinical skills and imaging findings. It is therefore vital that all relevant clinical information is known when performing and interpreting any radiological investigations. The referring clinician should be aware that not all positive imaging findings present on ultrasound or magnetic resonance imaging (MRI) are clinically important and that they can be found in an asymptomatic individual [11].

This section provides an overview of current radiological terminology with description and imaging findings and our diagnostic approach in processing the information from the history, clinical examination and imaging findings to formulate an optimal management plan.

The pubic symphysis represents the important cross-link between the strong adductor muscle complex and the anterior abdominal wall muscles and tendons. It is thus not unsurprising that the pubic bone often shows changes in sporting individuals and is often mislabeled as a diagnosis of osteitis pubis which is better reserved for females per partum where a more correct term of non-athletic osteitis pubis should be used (Fig. 17.2).

In the sporting athlete it is best practice to describe the bone marrow signal pattern observed on MRI with a common parasymphyseal bony oedema pattern, which is seen as an incidental finding with young footballers, but more diffuse bony oedema through a pubic body is a more positive finding.

The pubic symphysis is a secondary cartilaginous joint and with time it can develop a central cleft within its central fibrocartilage which is termed the primary cleft. This primary cleft may communicate with a secondary cleft which is an acquired cleft formed by separation of the short adductors (adductor brevis

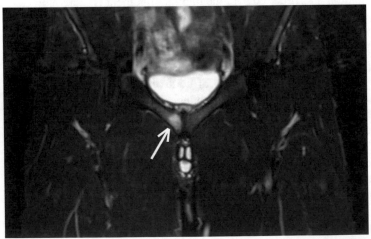

Fig. 17.2 MRI showing a footballer with a right pubic body stress response (*arrow*)

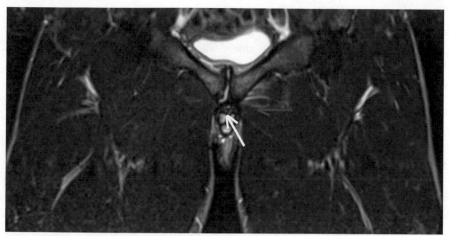

Fig. 17.3 MRI image showing a footballer with a right secondary cleft (*white arrow*) and a left adductor brevis grade 1 muscle strain (*red arrow*)

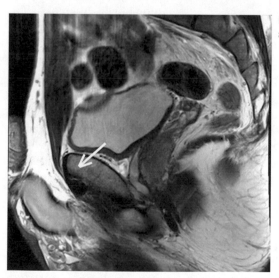

Fig. 17.4 MRI showing a right superior cleft sign (*arrow*)

and gracilis) from their bony attachments to the pubis. The secondary cleft is a description of partial tendon avulsion; it is a common finding in sporting athletes and it can be difficult to determine whether this represents an important finding that is responsible for the individual's current symptoms or an incidental finding from a previous injury (Fig. 17.3).

A further sign – the superior cleft sign – described where there is a cleft of high signal arising from the superior most tendinous attachment of the adductor longus to the pubic bone represents partial separation of the adductor longus and its aponeurosis from the superior pubic tubercle (Fig. 17.4).

These acute tears or adductor tendinous avulsions can be associated with bony oedema within the underlying bone.

Plain radiographs are useful to demonstrate gross degeneration or abnormalities of hip shape. More advanced imaging such as MR arthrography can reliably detect the presence of labral tears as well as early articular cartilage damage [25].

Ultrasound and MRI can be used to assess weakness of the posterior inguinal wall.

On MRI a hernial sac may also be visualized and strain scans can be performed but ultrasound is better suited in the assessment of the inguinal region for posterior inguinal wall weakness or disruption.

An ultrasound examination with graduated valsalva technique and forced valsalva are helpful in assessment for weakness of the posterior inguinal wall just medial to the deep inguinal ring; femoral hernia, although less common, can be also easily identified.

17.4   Management

17.4.1 Physiotherapy

Returning the athlete with groin pain back to sport is the aim of any physiotherapy programme.

To treat a sportsperson's injury the physiotherapist must recognize and be aware of the demands of the individual sport concerned especially once a more chronic PIPS condition is diagnosed.

Unfortunately, often the culture in sport is for the player not to report the pain until it is affecting their function and even then it does not limit their ability to train or play so they may well continue until the pain is too much; therefore, the actual true incidence of groin pain is unknown and it varies from sport to sport [26, 27].

A sports medicine team can often be judged on player availability and have to consequently spend time on prevention of a chronic injury but also accept that in sports acute injuries do occur.

There is very little evidence in the research, however, on the true causative factors which contribute to the exact etiology of PIPS depending upon a particular test. Much of the literature is focused on diagnosis, treatment and management.

It is though accepted in the literature that due to the multi-faceted nature of PIPS in the athlete an accurate diagnosis is more likely achieved through a multidisciplinary team approach [3]. Once an etiology is ascertained such as an adductor strain then preseason training and assessment can minimize the impact of the injury such as improving the adductor/abductor ratio [28]. In addition, Ekstrand and Gillquist found that preseason hip abduction range of motion was decreased in soccer players who subsequently sustained groin strains compared with uninjured players [29]. There is also randomized controlled trial evidence depicting how use of a specified physiotherapy programme has a greater chance of recovery and reducing the need for any surgical intervention [24].

Any rehabilitation generally concentrates on strengthening of the surrounding musculature and it should progress through static to functional exercise, through full range and last a minimum of 4 to 16 weeks. It is important that progression to the functional rehabilitation must not occur too early due to the pressure on the player to return. Rehabilitation can progress through outcome measures such as an asymptomatic isometric adductor squeeze, reduced range of internal rotation and/or a bent knee fall out. These outcomes can be used as useful monitoring tests to guide athlete's progression through each stage of the rehabilitation.

More recent evidence has reported on the presence of eccentric weakness of the adductor group while no isometric strength differences were observed. This may be another useful outcome to both measure and address in rehabilitation.

Centralization of the femoral head in the trochanter, like the shoulder, is achieved through both passive rigid structures like the congruence of the joint, labrum and capsule and the more dynamic structures like the soft tissue cuff made up of the adductors, gluteal complex and abdomen.

Effective treatment and management of the athlete with groin pain or indeed a prevention plan for an at-risk-athlete must identify abnormal motor patterning [28, 29].

The symptomatic athlete with groin pain will have a combination of weak gluteal muscles and adductors which are often in spasm as well as inhibition in the abdominal muscles that together as a group act as force couples to stabilize the lumbar, hip and pelvis complex to stabilize the femoral head.

Therefore, effective treatment of the athletic groin is not just about dealing with the pain-provoking structure but restoring the complex interaction of the soft tissue structures to centralize the femoral head.

Rehabilitation should last 4 weeks at the very least to restore correct movement patterns and if the patient's pain is controlled and their movement pattern is restored they may not need further intervention.

17.4.2 Surgery

Surgery has been at the forefront of treatment for patients with PIPS. It is still not clear as to what the preferred operation would be, whether open or laparoscopic, mesh or no mesh with a simple suture. The main techniques described include Lichtenstein, open minimal repair (OMR), transabdominal preperitoneal (TAPP) and transabdominal extraperitoneal (TEP) [6, 12, 30, 31]. All techniques have shown to provide an early return to sporting activity with the earlier work on open surgery using a specialized "darn" being slowly now superseded by minimal access techniques [30, 31]. A European survey of a large body of hernia surgeons has shown that the type of technique undertaken for repair was equally divided into mesh versus no mesh for open and for both minimal access techniques [32].

This study also concluded that there was no real consensus on the etiology of PIPS, with pain possibly arising from the inguinal canal, pubis symphysis and or the hip joint. The commonest finding in patients presenting with suspected PIPS is a weakened posterior wall indicating a conjoint tendon disruption [3]. Naturally any hip abnormality will not involve groin surgery, unless it is shown that there is dual pathology, which can occur in at least 20-50% of patients [4, 20]. The laparoscopic choice is increasingly becoming more common [33] although open minimal repair (OMR) still appears to have a role in surgical treatment for PIPS, especially as it has the advantage of no mesh/foreign body placement and an early return to sporting activity [12]. It appears, with this one exception, that the natural history of surgical repair for PIPS is taking the same route as inguinal hernia surgery with open Lichtenstein repair being replaced with more laparoscopic approaches [34]. A multicentre randomized controlled trial examining two common techniques (OMR and TEP) is presently ongoing (clinical trial no. NCT01876342) and should provide much-needed level I evidence as to which technique, if any, shows a better outcome in terms of an earlier return to sporting activity. Surgery for PIPS must, however, be accompanied by an active prehabilitation programme to try and improve core stability as this may prevent surgery [35]. However, if surgery is undertaken, a tailored rehabilitation programme to suit the needs of the individual with an early return to sporting activity is required. The nature of the rehabilitation will also depend upon the operation that has taken place, with open surgery possibly leading to a later return to sporting activity, although some reports have described return as early as two weeks especially with the OMR [12].

17.5   Conclusions

PIPS is a clinical entity involving the complex groin which will include all the surrounding structures. The hip, rectus abdominis aponeurosis, adductor complex as well as the pubic bone and inguinal canal are all possibly responsible either solely or in combination for the groin pain seen in athletes. Despite the complex etiology the correct pathology can be identified with a careful history, examination findings and the relevant investigations, as described above. For high-performing athletes a multidisciplinary approach is the preferred manner in which all such patients should be managed.

References

1. Moeller JL (2007) Sportsman's hernia. Curr Sports Med Rep 6:111–114
2. Holmich P, Renstrom PA (2007) Long-standing groin pain in sportspeople falls into three primary patterns, a "clinical entity" approach: a prospective study of 207 patients. Br J Sports Med 41:247–252

3. Sheen AJ, Stephenson B, Lloyd DM et al (2014) Treatment of the sportsman's groin: British Hernia Society's 2014 position statement based on the Manchester Consensus Conference. Br J Sports Med 48:1079–1087
4. Campanelli G (2010) Pubic inguinal pain syndrome: the so-called sports hernia. Hernia 14:1–4
5. Weir A, Brukner P, Delahunt E et al (2015) Doha agreement meeting on terminology and definitions in groin pain in athletes. Br J Sports Med 49:768–774
6. Mann CD, Sutton CD, Garcea G et al (2009) The inguinal release procedure for groin pain: initial experience in 73 sportsmen/women. Br J Sports Med 43:579–583
7. Orchard J, Read JW, Verall GM et al (2000) Patho-physiology of chronic groin pain in the athlete. Int Sports Med J 1:1–20
8. Hackney RG (1993) The sports hernia: a cause of chronic groin pain. Br J Sports Med 27:58–62
9. Swan KG Jr, Wolcott M (2007) The athletic hernia: a systematic review. Clin Orthop Relat Res 455:78–87
10. Gilmore J (1998) Groin pain in the soccer athlete: fact, fiction, and treatment. Clin Sports Med 17:787–793
11. Robinson P, Grainger AJ, Hensor EMA et al (2015) Do MRI and ultrasound of the anterior pelvis correlate with, or predict, young football players' clinical findings? A 4-year prospective study of elite academy soccer players. Br J Sports Med 49:176–182
12. Muschaweck U, Berger L (2010) Minimal repair technique of sportsmen's groin: an innovative open-suture repair to treat chronic inguinal pain. Hernia 14:27–33
13. Nicholson J, Scott M (2012) Conjoint tendon disruption: redefining and recognizing "Gilmore's groin" a review of 1200 cases. Hernia 16:143–240
14. Pun S, Kumar D, Lane N (2015) Femoroacetabular impingement. Arthritis & Reumatology: 67:17–27
15. Jaberi FM, Parvizi J (2007) Hip pain in young adults: femoroacetabular impingement. J Arthroplasty 22(Suppl 3):37–42
16. Beck M, Kalhor M, Leunig M et al (2005) Hip morphology influences the pattern of damage to the acetabular cartilage: femoroacetabular impingement as a cause of early osteoarthritis of the hip. J Bone Joint Surg Br 87:1012–1018
17. Ganz R, Parvizi J, Beck M et al (2003) Femoroacetabular impingement: a cause for osteoarthritis of the hip. Clin Orthop Relat Res 417:112–120
18. Agricola R, Bessems JH, Ginai AZ et al (2012) The development of Cam-type deformity in adolescent and young male soccer players. Am J Sports Med 40:1099–1106
19. Colen S, Van den Bekerom MP, Bellemans J et al (2010) Comparison of intra-articular injections of hyaluronic acid and corticosteroid in the treatment of osteoarthritis of the hip in comparison with intra-articular injections of bupivacaine. Design of a prospective, randomized, controlled study with blinding of the patients and outcome assessors. BMC Musculoskelet Disord 11:264
20. Bisciotti GN, Auci A, Di Marzo F et al (2015) Groin pain syndrome: an association of different pathologies and a case presentation. Muscles Ligaments Tendons J 5:214–222
21. Naal FD, Dalla Riva F, Wuerz TH et al (2015) Sonographic prevalence of groin hernias and adductor tendinopathy in patients with femoroacetabular impingement. Am J Sports Med 43:2146–2151
22. Tegner Y Lorentzon R (1991) Ice hockey injuries: incidence, nature and causes. Brit J Sports Med 25:87–89
23. Renstrom P Peterson L (1980) Groin injuries in athletes. Brit J Sports Med 14:30–36
24. Holmich P, Uhrskou P, Ulnits L et al (1999) Effectiveness of active physical training as treatment for long-standing adductor-related groin pain in athletes: randomised trial. Lancet 353:439–443
25. Domayer SE, Ziebarth K, Chan J et al (2011) Femoroacetabular cam-type impingement: diagnostic sensitivity and specificity of radiographic views compared to radial MRI. Eur J Radiol: 80:805–810

26. Molsa J, Airaksinen O, Nasman O et al (1997) Ice hockey injuries in Finland. A prospective epidemiologic study. Am J Sports Med 25:495–499
27. Nielsen AB, Yde J (1989) Epidemiology and traumatology of injuries in soccer. Am J Sports Med 17:803–807
28. Tyler TF, Nicholas SJ, Campbell RJ et al (2001) The association of hip strength and flexibility with the incidence of adductor muscle strains in professional ice hockey players. Am J Sports Med 29:124–128
29. Ekstrand J, Gillquist J (1983) The avoidability of soccer injuries. Int J Sports Med 4:124–128
30. Gilmore OJA (1991) Gilmore's groin: ten years experience of groin disruption – a previously unsolved problem in sportsmen. Sports Med Soft Tissue Trauma 3:12–14
31. Paajanen H, Brinck T, Hermunen H et al (2011) Laparoscopic surgery for chronic groin pain in athletes is more effective than nonoperative treatment: a randomised clinical trial with magnetic resonance imaging of 60 patients with sportsman's hernia (athletic pubalgia). Surgery 150:99–107
32. Kingston JA, Jegatheeswaran S, Macutkiewicz C (2014) A European survey on the aetiology, investigation and management of the 'sportsman's groin'. Hernia 18:803–810
33. Susmallian S, Ezri T, Elis M et al (2004) Laparoscopic repair of 'sportsman's hernia' in soccer players as treatment of chronic inguinal pain. Med Sci Monit 10: CR52–54
34. Sheen AJ, Paajanen H (2015) The next step towards rational treatment for 'The sportsman' groin'. Br J Sports Med 49:764–765
35. Hölmich P, Larsen K, Krogsgaard K et al (2010) Exercise program for prevention of groin pain in football players: a cluster-randomised trial. Scand J Med Sci Sports 20:814–821

Obscure Groin Pain in Women

18

Shirin Towfigh

18.1 History of the Hidden Hernia

The concept of hidden hernias was first introduced in the 1970s by two separately interested surgeons from the United States: William Webb from Alabama and Jack Herrington from Wisconsin. They each noticed that women were presenting with symptoms suggestive of inguinal hernia, however the surgeons had a hard time diagnosing a hernia on physical examination. Their patients reported intermittent pain along the inguinal canal that was related to physical activity. However, the physical examination was essentially normal and "without detectable impulse".

Webb reported his experience with 12 women who had symptomatic inguinal hernias without diagnostic examination findings. Physical examination was mostly normal. He offered them an exploration based on their history alone. They presented similar to most other symptomatic inguinal hernias: groin pain radiating along the inguinal canal. He found that these women typically had small indirect inguinal hernias with preperitoneal fat content only. There was no hernia sac. Repair was successful in all the patients, with resolution of their preoperative pain.

Over a 5-year period of time, Herrington operated on 13 such patients (8% of his practice), all of whom were also women. They suffered with groin pain of undiagnosed etiology. Mean age was 20 years (15-45). Most had undergone a wide range of gastrointestinal, urologic, and gynecologic workups. Operative findings were of the typical indirect inguinal hernia and most had a peritoneal sac. At 10 months follow-up, 10 (77%) patients had a cure of their symptoms after open inguinal hernia repair and 3 patients had significant improvement. He referred to these as "female occult inguinal hernias", and urged their early diagnosis, as hernia repair was curative.

S. Towfigh (✉)
Beverly Hills Hernia Center, Cedars-Sinai Medical Center, Department of Surgery
Beverly Hills, California, USA
email: drtowfigh@beverlyhillsherniacenter.com

G. Campanelli (Ed), *Inguinal Hernia Surgery*,
Updates in Surgery
DOI: 10.1007/978-88-470-3947-6_18, © Springer-Verlag Italia 2017

The concept of the non-palpable, symptomatic, occult or hidden hernia did not become popular despite these ground breaking reports. Textbooks continued to report 25% lifetime risk of inguinal hernias among males and only 2% risk among females. It wasn't until Bendavid's textbook of *Abdominal Wall Hernias* that this topic was readdressed in the 21st century.

Similar to their predecessors, Spangen and Smedberg reported on 180 women in an 18-year span with 192 occult hernias. Most were found to have typical inguinal hernias with peritoneal sac. However, 57 (30%) had inguinal hernias with preperitoneal fat content only and no peritoneal extension within the inguinal canal. They had successful outcomes after hernia repair, with relief of preoperative symptoms in 89% of patients, with mean 20 (1-60) months follow-up.

18.2   Anatomical Explanation for the Hidden Hernia

Women naturally have a narrower inguinal canal than men. Essentially, it contains a thin round ligament and perhaps the genital branch of the genitofemoral nerve. Conversely, males begin with a naturally wider inguinal canal that houses the spermatic cord. Meanwhile, the female pelvis is broader and shallower. As a result, the insertion of the internal oblique and transversus abdominis muscles is broader along Cooper's ligament and further onto the rectus muscle. Also, the round ligament pierces the abdominal wall more laterally and follows a more oblique path within the inguinal canal. Lastly, the natural forces from gravity and from internal abdominal pressure are distributed more evenly along the pelvic floor, as compared to that in the narrow pelvis of men.

As a result, women tend not to present with wide palpable defects or significant bulging from their hernia. Instead, they present with groin pain, sometimes with the very smallest amount of preperitoneal fat entering the narrow inguinal canal.

On physical examination, men typically have a palpable if not visible bulge. When standing, an impulse may be generated by Valsalva or cough. Using the redundancy of the scrotal skin, the spermatic cord can be followed toward the external ring and the rest of the pelvic floor in this region can be directly palpated. In women, there is no direct access to the external ring and the inguinal canal contents. Palpation is made directly over the inguinal canal at the level of the skin. Any hernia must be noted through the layers of skin, soft tissue, and external oblique aponeurosis. If a vaginal examination is performed, the examiner can sometimes detect a mass via the vaginal sidewall. This is another reason for the occult non-palpable hernia.

18.3   Symptoms in Women

Hernias among women tend to present with a wide variety of symptoms. As many of these symptoms are not similar to those typical of men, it can delay their diagnosis. In my practice, I have shown that the typical hernia was diagnosed by me after 20 weeks of presentation. Those with hidden hernias averaged 96 weeks of symptoms. Typically, the dominant symptoms for hernias among women are activity-related, such as pain with lifting heavy objects. Normal daily routines that cause increased pressure onto the inguinal canal may also cause pain, such as prolonged sitting, prolonged standing, bending. The pain is often worse at the end of the day. Pain may also be distributed along the distribution of the ilioinguinal and genital nerves, and this can be misinterpreted as primary neuropathic pain. In my experience, some of these patients undergo local nerve block to address the neuropathic pain. If a hernia is the cause of the neuropathic type pain, I have noted that patients report an increase in their groin pain after the nerve block, whereas a nerve block should improve pain in the case of a true primary nerve injury without a hernia.

Though men do not typically present with pain as their primary complaint from their inguinal hernia, such is not the trend with women. Among women, groin pain is often the first presenting symptom. Many surgeons are trained to believe that pain alone cannot be due to an inguinal hernia. This may be true among most male patients; it is not the case in women. As a result, many women are labelled as having chronic pelvic pain, and inguinal hernia is not considered to be the cause of their groin pain.

As we already know, smaller hernia defects tend to present with more pain and less bulging, whereas larger hernia defects tend to present with a bulge without as much pain. So it may be the case that women with inguinal hernias, many of which are hidden hernias, present with pain as their original symptom, and not with a palpable bulge. The patient may complain of radiating pain, which I found to be seen among almost half (48%) of my patients (Table 18.1). This includes pain radiating pain from the groin into the vagina, to the upper inner thigh, to the anterior thigh – but never below the level of the knee – and/or wrapping around laterally toward the hip and back. In my experience, 20% of patients have associated lower back pain that resolves after hernia repair. Such patients may be misdiagnosed with spinal pathology. Notably, patients with lower back pain do not have groin pain, with the exception of sacroiliitis, which can cause pain radiating from the back to the groin and upper inner thigh.

Also, 39% of my female patients have radiating pain into the vagina (Table 18.1). This is analogous to the pain radiating to the base of penis and/or testicle in men. Such a complaint can trigger a gynecologic workup of obscure diagnoses such as vulvodynia, pudendal neuralgia, and chronic pelvic pain. These diagnoses often have complex syndromes that are not seen among patients with inguinal hernia.

Symptoms unique to women include pain during menses. In my practice, 25% of women with symptomatic inguinal hernias report exacerbation of their symptoms during their menses (Table 18.1). This is considered to be due to fluctuations in hormones. As estrogen levels plummet at the onset of menstruation, pain levels increase. This phenomenon has been shown in multiple other disease processes, including joint disorders, autoimmune disorders, and gastrointestinal diseases. In such cases, women are commonly worked up for endometriosis, which is a cyclical disease. Unlike endometriosis, hernias are not pain-free in between menstrual periods.

In women, hernias can be painful during sexual intercourse as well as with orgasm. The reason for pain with intercourse is often a simple phenomenon of direct contact and pressure on the groin. Similarly, vaginal penetration can cause pain by direct pressure onto the external ring, which we noted earlier could be palpable transvaginally. Pain with orgasm is considered to be due to pelvic floor contraction against a full inguinal canal.

Table 18.1 Key history and examination findings predictive of female symptomatic occult inguinal hernia, with expected outcomes after hernia repair

Symptoms	Prevalence
Pain as primary symptom	87%
Radiating quality to the groin pain	48%
– Radiating pain to the vagina	39%
– Radiating pain to lower back	20%
Worse with menses	25%
Pain during intercourse	
Pain with orgasm	
Examination Findings	
Point tenderness over deep internal ring	96–100%
Hyperalgesia along ilioinguinal nerve	63%
Subtle fullness overlying inguinal canal	52%
Pelvic floor spasm	
Operative Findings	
Preperitoneal fat only, no hernia sac	>30%
Significant improvement in preoperative symptoms after hernia repair	78–87%

18.4   Subtle Physical Examination Findings

The concept of the occult inguinal hernia is based on the finding of a symptomatic inguinal hernia without obvious findings on physical examination. This includes no visible bulge and no detectable impulse. For example, a cough or Valsalva will typically not generate a bulging mass on external examination in this population. That said, in my experience, 96% of these patients have point tenderness at the level of the internal ring upon direct pressure. Spangen similarly reported 100% with point tenderness overlying the deep internal ring upon Valsalva. He also reported 63% with hyperalgesia along the ilioinguinal nerve distribution (Table 18.1).

With a very sensitive touch, the examiner can feel a subtle fullness in the area overlying the deep internal ring among those with a symptomatic hidden hernia. I have noted this in 52% of my patients with symptomatic occult inguinal hernias. This represents content and probably inflammation in the area of the inguinal canal. It is also often tender over the same area. If this area of vague fullness correlates with the area of pain, which correlates with the area over the deep internal ring, we have shown this to be the most sensitive predictor of a hidden hernia (Fig. 18.1).

Many women are first evaluated for their groin pain by their gynecologist. Pelvic exam can be painful on the side of the inguinal hernia. There may be finding of pelvic floor spasm as well. Some patients are referred to pelvic floor physical therapy for this reason. In my experience, I have noted that such therapy

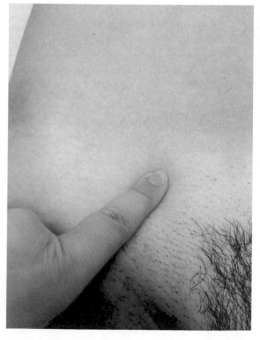

Fig. 18.1 Area of maximal tenderness and vague fullness notable in patients with symptomatic occult inguinal hernias. This area is approximately half-way between the anterior superior iliac crest and pubic tubercle on each side

exacerbates the patient's pain if she has an inguinal hernia and not primary pelvic floor dysfunction. Also, I have noted that the pelvic floor spasm resolves after successful inguinal hernia repair.

Thus, I have come to the conclusion that inguinal hernias can cause pelvic floor spasm in women. This results in the sequelae seen with this entity, including chronic pelvic pain, pain with sexual intercourse, urinary frequency, feeling of pain or pressure at the vagina or rectum. The workup and treatment can be highly varied and patients may be misdiagnosed with interstitial cystitis or pelvic floor dysfunction. These disorders are multifactorial and are defined by a series of objective findings, such as with cystoscopy or dynamic pelvic imaging, respectively. The workup would be normal in those with inguinal hernia.

18.5   Conclusions

Women can have inguinal hernias and it is much more prevalent than we are led to believe historically. Women are more likely than men to present with groin pain without bulging mass, hence the term female occult inguinal hernia or hidden hernia. Carefully listening to the patient will allow the examiner to identify key details in their history that are suggestive of inguinal hernia. The most sensitive examination finding is that of point tenderness over the area of the deep internal ring. Operative findings may show preperitoneal fat content only, without peritoneal extension.

As more attention is placed on this entity, more women will be diagnosed, without delay, with a potential for improvement in their quality of life.

Suggested Readings

Fodor PB, Webb WA (1971) Indirect inguinal hernia in the female with no palpable sac. South Med J 64:15

Herrington JK (1975) Occult inguinal hernia in the female. Ann Surg 181:481-483

Neumayer L, Towfigh S (2013) Inguinal hernia. In: Cameron JL, Cameron AM (eds) Current surgical therapy, 11th edn. Elsevier, New York, pp 531-536

Rutkow IM (1998) Epidemiologic, economic, and sociologic aspects of hernia surgery in the United States in the 1990s. Surg Clin N Am 78:941-951, v-vi

Saad CA, Kim DS, Solnik MJ, Towfigh S (2015) Inguinal hernia as a cause of chronic pelvic pain: a key sign to make the diagnosis. Obst Gyn 125:70S

Spangen L, Smedberg SGG (2001) Nonpalpable inguinal hernia in women. In: Bendavid R, Abrahamson J, Arregui ME et al (eds) Abdominal wall hernias. Springer, New York, pp 625-629

Zarrinkhoo E, Towfigh S, Miller J (2015) Hidden hernias as a cause of chronic pelvic pain. Hernia 19:S73-S76

Future Perspectives on Complications in Inguinal Hernia Repair

19

René H. Fortelny and Alexander H. Petter-Puchner

19.1 Introduction

Inguinal hernia research and repair has become an increasingly complex surgical field. The past two decades have seen the acceptance of meshes as standard of care, the development of atraumatic fixation devices, the introduction of biologic implants and the implementation of tissue-engineered synthetic absorbable matrices in the clinical setting. Single-incision procedures reflect the progress of surgical procedures.

Today, bioabsorbable synthetic meshes are enthusiastically promoted as a possible replacement for biologic meshes delivering reproducible results without unpredictable adverse effects. Generally, the hope is high that the combination of tissue-engineered scaffolds with cell therapies will eventually allow functional repair.

The pace of these developments is truly breathtaking. However, the translation to benefits for patients remains frequently disputed. Looking at the literature on contemporary biologic meshes, these were initially presented as a solution to most major concerns in hernia repair (e.g., reconstruction, use in contaminated wound fields, superior biocompatibility). Today, one has to admit that these hopes have not materialized. To the contrary, biologic collagen implants seem to provoke unpredictable foreign body reactions and are prone to slow integration, which can lead to serious complications. Therefore, the story of biologic meshes serves as an example of how to deal with complications with new products in hernia surgery in the future.

In this chapter, three areas of complications will be defined and linked to promising developments in the field (Table 19.1):

R.H. Fortelny (✉)
Department of General, Visceral and Oncological Surgery, Wilhelminen Spital
Vienna, Austria
e-mail: rene.fortelny@wienkav.at

G. Campanelli (Ed), *Inguinal Hernia Surgery,*
Updates in Surgery
DOI: 10.1007/978-88-470-3947-6_19, © Springer-Verlag Italia 2017

Table 19.1 Possible future complications in inguinal hernia repair

Complication	Possible areas of concern in the future
Mesh-related	Bioabsorbable synthetic mesh: recurrences, seroma?
Fixation-related	Cyanoacrylates meshes Self-gripping meshes Non fixation: long-term recurrence rate
Procedure-related	SIL repair: port site incisional hernia
	Robotic hernia repair ??
Biotechnological	Cellular therapies: rejection, sepsis, viability New synthetic and biologic matrices: foreign body reaction, unpredictable behavior (resorption, integration)

SIL, single-incision laparoscopic.

- *mesh-related* and *fixation-related* complications
- *procedure-related* complications
- *biotechnological* complications

19.2 Mesh-related Complications

19.2.1 Biologic Meshes

It is highly unlikely that biologic meshes will play a relevant role in inguinal hernia repair in the future. In consequence, it should be sufficient to point out that there is no clinical evidence for superiority over synthetic meshes in inguinal hernia repair or any other indication. A recent publication in the ANZ Journal of Surgery demonstrated that biologic inguinal hernia repair was associated with longer operation times and more seroma formation compared to standard mesh repair [1].

19.2.2 Bioabsorbable Synthetic Meshes

A new class of synthetic mesh was introduced to the market in the recent past, namely bioabsorbable implants, such as BioA (polyglycolic acid/trimethylene carbonate), TIGR (polylactic and polyglycolic acid) and Phasix (poly-4-hydroxybutyrate). Potential advantages include rapid integration and a mild foreign body reaction compared to biologic meshes. Compared to the other above mentioned meshes, the BioA represents a 3D matrix rather than a 2D mesh layer. TIGR and Phasix are more conventional in design, but all three share the feature of being resorbed in 9 to 24 months after implantation. Our study group could demonstrate that the BioA actually reinforces the abdominal wall by eliciting a robust scar formation, yielding reticular collagen formation. If this is also achieved by the other competitors has, to the best of our knowledge, not been investigated in detail yet. Considering the ongoing debate about genetic and epigenetic factors influencing hernia formation, it is totally unclear if resorbable meshes could lead to an increased rate of recurrences.

This issue will become even more important as a variety of synthetic, resorbable meshes will enter the market in the near future. Furthermore, it must be emphasized that the resorption process of these implants (most of them polyglycolic/polylactic acid derivatives) could lead to seroma formation or prolonged local inflammation. Because bioabsorbable, synthetic meshes have been presented as direct competitors of collagen matrices, many surgeons are eager to use them in contaminated wound fields. The first study using BioA in contaminated fields (CDC class 2 and 3 [2]) with promising results was published recently [3]. The future will show how these new meshes will perform in other than clean wounds (e.g., after resection of incarcerated bowel).

19.2.3 Polypropylene and Polyester Meshes

Although polypropylene and polyester meshes are the most commonly used implants in hernia repair and are usually well tolerated, it is currently unclear how these polymers behave in terms of aging and mechanical breakdown. If implanted in young adults, meshes will have to perform for up to seven decades considering the life expectancy in developed countries. There is at least some evidence that differences between polypropylene and polyester can be found [4]. However, this question must be elucidated in more detail in the future.

19.3 Fixation-related Complications

While there is an impressive safety record for biologic sealants (e.g., fibrin sealant such as Tisseel/Tissucol, Baxter, Round Lake, USA) [5], the long-term effects of other atraumatic fixation methods are fully unknown. The application of cyanoacrylates is tempting because of quick adhesion and easy use. It has repeatedly been demonstrated that cyanoacrylates impair tissue integration [6], can exert serious damage to instruments and are inadequate for being sprayed in a uniform layer. Although it is true that the clinical importance of these observations has not yet been verified, the progress with cyanoacrylates for mesh fixation in inguinal hernia repair should be critically followed over the next years.

The analysis of recurrence rates and local pain sensation will also be worthwhile for self-gripping meshes, like Covidien-Medtronic's Progrip mesh [7]. While the concept is intriguing and the likelihood of complications is low, it is important to know that the resorption rate of the polylactic acid (PLA) grips seem to vary between individuals [8]. If and how this could translate to mesh dislocation and prolonged foreign body reaction is again unclear.

The major topic in the area of fixation-related complications could be the consequences of non-fixation. Non-fixation of meshes is nothing new in totally extra-peritoneal (TEP) repair and has become an accepted alternative in transabdominal preperitoneal (TAPP) repair as well [9]. In awareness of recent modifications in the guidelines [10] embracing non-fixation in laparoscopic inguinal hernia repair, it must be emphasized that the long-term impact on recurrence rates cannot be fully appreciated yet. In other words, more randomized controlled trials will be needed to falsify the hypothesis that non-fixation is generally unproblematic.

19.4   Procedure-related Complications

Refined operating techniques and sophisticated materials have elevated the standard of care to a high level. Procedure-related complications usually arise when techniques are changing because of innovations in instruments or new scientific insights. In most cases it will be a combination of both, e.g., it was the insight that postoperative pain could be reduced by atraumatic fixation that led to the development of specialized fibrin sealants and application devices; the reported complication was a rise of the incidence of seromas in TAPP, because surgeons initially used too much sealant. Today and in the future the main procedural changes are represented by single-incision laparoscopic (SIL) repairs [11] and the introduction of robotics to hernia repair.

The possibility of creating port-site incisional hernias after SIL procedures will remain a passionately disputed issue. The meticulous preparation of fascial edges and closure with slow, non-resorbable running suture in small bite technique is essential and any deviation will invariably lead to a phenomenon the authors call "hernia shift" (i.e., closure of a preexistent hernia with the SIL technique resulting in a port-site hernia) [12].

The benefits, risks and complications associated with robotic hernia surgery need to be weighed and assessed in the future [13]. More and more hospitals acquire robots and, as they become cheaper and more versatile, they will be more frequently used in standard procedures such as hernia repair. Currently, the data are scarce and it is too early to define or predict the relevant areas of concern.

In any case, the education and specific training of surgeons, supporting manual skills and enabling profound understanding of underlying problems, can help to avoid procedure-related complications.

19.5   Biotechnological Complications

This section shall summarize the risk of humoral and cellular therapies, as well as inflammatory and immunologic responses to biologic and synthetic matrices. An example of complications of cellular therapies was rejection of allogenic cell transplants (although not a feasible treatment option due to regulatory issues) or sepsis as a sequel of premature cell death of autologous cells (e.g., when the cell grafts are not sufficiently vascularized). A biotechnological complication of implants could already be observed in the massive tissue reaction to cross-linked collagen and non-cross-linked implants. The *a priori* working hypothesis that a collagen matrix must be better tolerated by the human organism was simply wrong and contradicted by granuloma formation (to cross-linked) and rapid fragmentation (of non-cross-linked) biologic meshes [14]. It is almost certain that similar experiences will be made in future with other new materials and a clear identification of the problem will be mandatory to protect our patients. The development of autologous stem cell therapy to enhance tissue integration and prevent adhesion formation and, secondly, to improve functionality in abdominal wall repair will be seen in the future and will demand a careful balance of desirable progress and caution [15].

19.6   Conclusions

Looking closely at the past and present of inguinal hernia repair helps to anticipate future problems and complications by tailoring the procedure to the patient in terms of operation technique and choice of mesh material. To define and predict the individual risk of complication and recurrence we need further basic experimental research and data from hernia registries [16].

The advent of cellular therapies and the momentum that tissue engineering concepts are starting to develop in hernia repair demand the will and mindfulness of researchers and clinicians alike to perform one step after the other. The lessons learned from biologic meshes should be clear. It serves nobody in the field to let hopes and expectations blur the view on what is actually going on. Even when bearing these experiences in mind, seeing what is actually going on is a difficult task for so many contributions to the field every day. Learning from others will probably be the best way to ensure that our patients are safe and our endeavors successful.

References

1. Fang Z, Ren F, Zhou J, Tian J (2015) Biologic mesh versus synthetic mesh in open inguinal hernia repair: system review and meta-analysis. ANZ J Surg 85:910–916
2. Mangram AJ, Horan TC, Pearson ML et al (1999) Guideline for prevention of surgical site infection. Hospital Infection Control Practices Advisory Committee. Infect Control Hosp Epidemiol 20:250–278
3. Rosen MJ, Bauer JJ, Harmaty M et al (2016) Multicenter, prospective, longitudinal study of the recurrence, surgical site infection, and quality of life after contaminated ventral hernia repair using biosynthetic absorbable mesh: the COBRA Study. Ann Surg [Epub ahead of print] doi:10.1097/SLA.0000000000001601

4. Cozad MJ, Grant DA, Bachman SL et al (2010) Materials characterization of explanted polypropylene, polyethylene terephthalate, and expanded polytetrafluoroethylene composites: spectral and thermal analysis. J Biomed Mater Res B Appl Biomater 94:455–462

5. Fortelny RH, Petter-Puchner AH, Glaser KS, Redl H (2012) Use of fibrin sealant (Tisseel/Tissucol) in hernia repair: a systematic review. Surg Endosc 26:1803–1812

6. Fortelny RH, Petter-Puchner AH, Walder N (2007) Cyanoacrylate tissue sealant impairs tissue integration of macroporous mesh in experimental hernia repair. Surg Endosc 21:1781–1785

7. Zhang C, Li F, Zhang H et al (2013) Self-gripping versus sutured mesh for inguinal hernia repair: a systematic review and meta-analysis of current literature. J Surg Res 185:653–660

8. Gruber-Blum S, Riepl N, Brand J et al (2014) A comparison of Progrip and Adhesix self-adhering hernia meshes in an onlay model in the rat. Hernia18:761–769

9. Mayer F, Niebuhr H, Lechner M et al (2016) When is mesh fixation in TAPP-repair of primary inguinal hernia repair necessary? The register-based analysis of 11,230 cases. Surg Endosc [Epub ahead of print] doi:10.1007/s00464-016-4754-8

10. Bittner R, Montgomery MA, Arregui E et al (2015) Update of guidelines on laparoscopic (TAPP) and endoscopic (TEP) treatment of inguinal hernia. Surg Endosc 29:289–321

11. Petter-Puchner AH, Brunner W, Gruber-Blum S et al (2014) A systematic review of hernia surgery in SIL (single-incision laparoscopy) technique. Eur Surg 46:113–117

12. Antoniou SA, Morales-Conde S, Antoniou GA et al (2016) Single-incision laparoscopic surgery through the umbilicus is associated with a higher incidence of trocar-site hernia than conventional laparoscopy: a meta-analysis of randomized controlled trials. Hernia 20:1–10

13. Vorst AL, Kaoutzanis C, Carbonell AM, Franz MG (2015) Evolution and advances in laparoscopic ventral and incisional hernia repair. World J Gastrointest Surg 7:293–305

14. Petter-Puchner AH, Fortelny RH (2015) The heart of darkness. Hernia 19:195–196

15. Petter-Puchner AH, Fortelny RH, Gruber-Blum S et al (2015) The future of stem cell therapy in hernia and abdominal wall repair. Hernia 19:25–31

16. Köckerling F, Bittner R, Jacob DA et al (2015) TEP versus TAPP: comparison of the perioperative outcome in 17,587 patients with a primary unilateral inguinal hernia. Surg Endosc 29:3750–3760

Treatment Cost Reimbursement from the Healthcare Systems

20

Dalila Patrizia Greco, Fabio Amatucci, and Giovanni Andrea Padula

20.1 Reimbursement

It is difficult to ensure an effective reimbursement mechanism in the delivery of healthcare without the government system of the tariff scheme. This system generates a price for a particular service or treatment, differentiating each case according to the complexity of patient treatments (casemix) and use of resources, both human and technological, including medical devices and pharmaceutical products.

This type of reimbursement system reduces potential inappropriate activity [1, 2] and incentivizes the development of patient care quality [3], so providers have the resources and flexibility to deliver the best possible healthcare services. In the current scenario of technological innovation and progressively ageing population, the Italian tariff scheme (TUC, Tariffa Unica Convenzionale) lacks the ability to reflect the real cost of providing healthcare.

20.2 Healthcare System

Public health is considered a primary asset in any country [3] and its protection is extensive to a greater or lesser level. The progressively ageing population, improvements in social conditions and advances in medical knowledge combined with technological progress are recognized as being the main causes of two situations. There is an increase in demand for healthcare services, caused by both the ageing population and the increased standards of living. On the other hand, there is the need to implement healthcare management [3, 4] because the cost of

D.P. Greco (✉)
Day and Week Surgery Unit, Multi Specialist Surgery Department, ASST Grande Ospedale Metropolitano Niguarda,
Milan, Italy
e-mail: dalila.greco@ospedaleniguarda.it

G. Campanelli (Ed), *Inguinal Hernia Surgery,*
Updates in Surgery
DOI: 10.1007/978-88-470-3947-6_20, © Springer-Verlag Italia 2017

Table 20.1 Healthcare funding systems

BISMARCK MODEL	Almost universal healthcare system based on mandatory social insurances. There are several funding sources such as social contributions and taxes to cover healthcare services/treatments. To leave the social healthcare system, citizens could buy a private healthcare insurance.
Country	**Funding characteristics**
Austria: Bismarck	Social insurances (social contribution).
Belgium: Bismarck	Social insurances (social contribution). There are various types of social insurances and citizens have the right to choose health insurance.
East Europe: Bismarck	Single social insurance managed by the State.
France: impure Bismarck	Mandatory social insurances: public or private health insurance funds.
Germany: Bismarck	Solidaristic System. Social protection and insurance circuit covers 86.9%, an additional 2.4 % receives state coverage, 11% of the population opt for a form of private insurance coverage.
Netherlands: atypical Bismarck	Mandatory health insurance. Citizens have the right to choose health insurance and they are free to change insurance company once a year.
BEVERIDGE MODEL	Establishment of a national health service based on universal coverage and mainly, if not exclusively, financed by general taxation (national or local). Private insurances overlap the public coverage, offering additional guarantees such as freedom of choice and time of access to the benefits or to the services not covered by NHS (National Health System).
Country	**Funding characteristics**
Denmark/Sweden/ Finland: Beveridge	NHS - Decentralized system: the commitment to provide services is mainly Beveridge in the hands of local authorities.
Greece: Beveridge	NHS - ESY "Ethniko Systima Ygeias" – with the presence of a complex network of social insurance of illness (ASM).
Ireland: Beveridge	NHS - The right to healthcare benefits is recognized only based on resident status and not on the payment of contributions. The 1st category is "absolutely entitled" (Medical Card); the 2nd category does not enjoy some free services but it has the right to treatment and to stay in public hospitals at no charge.
Italy: Beveridge	NHS - The level of resources is determined annually at a central level by Regional general taxation. Citizens have to contribute by co-payment (ticket), patients with chronic diseases or with social hardship are relieved.
Portugal: Beveridge	The NHS is managed, regulated and planned at a central level; although health service delivery is structured on a regional level. Universal coverage is mostly cost-free at the point of care.

(cont.) →

Table 20.1 *(continued)*

Spain: Beveridge	The NHS has an open access and predominant role as a public service. Free level, central, local and Autonomous Communities.
United Kingdom: hybrid Beveridge	NHS - The funding sources are mainly public (83%) through taxation and VHI (Voluntary Health Insurance) covers 3%, out-of-pocket payment (14%).
United States: neither Beveridge, nor Bismarck	Private insurances (companies, individuals) 78%; large public programs (Medicaid, Medicare, SCHIP) 21%; sum of both the sources 1%.

healthcare cannot be increased. This cost is always covered by the user through general taxation, self-financing through insurance, health insurance funds or out of pocket payments [5].

Healthcare systems should be comparable in order to create both a basis for evaluation and a benchmarking system necessary to assess appropriateness and efficiency of the system. To achieve this goal, some countries have adopted a philosophy of reimbursement, which aims to split healthcare services into clusters of patients defined as homogenous [6–8]. In particular, homogenous is referred to a cluster of patients who receive "standard" surgical, medical, or rehabilitative care based on the diagnosis and that is differentiated according to age group into child or adult care [9, 10]. An international comparison of the different approaches to reimbursement in some European and extra-European health systems is shown in Table 20.1, while Table 20.2 shows the reimbursement mechanisms adopted in the same countries [8–13]

Since the existing reimbursement mechanism in Italy is based on the diagnostic-related groups (DRGs) system [13], we have focused our evaluation on this logic/categorization of reimbursement.

Our analysis is based on DRG 161–163 which include inguinal hernia surgery that are among the group of abdominal wall surgery procedures DRG 159–163. DRG 161–163 include procedures for inguinal/femoral hernia with or without complications in childhood and adulthood, while DRG 159–160 include the remaining abdominal wall surgeries: umbilical hernia, incisional hernia, diastasis recti. More specifically, as regards inguinal hernia surgery, Table 20.3 shows the Italian distribution of the cases reimbursed with regard to the four abovementioned DRG, for each region in the first half of 2015.

Hernioplasty is performed with different surgical techniques not properly described by the codes 53.00 to 53.39. The same problem is associated with DRG 159–160 (laparoplasty), whose procedures are included in codes 53.4 to 53.9. Sometimes there is a need to combine surgical procedures on abdominal viscera and the same DRG reimburses simple and complex procedures. Existing reimbursement mechanisms do not take into account the clinical characteristics of the services they are paying for. In fact, a single cluster includes procedures such

Table 20.2 Providers' reimbursement systems

Budget	A total constraint is established on the amount of resources available for the single provider. It is mainly used by the "Beveridge systems", sometimes it is weighted per capita share. In the "Bismarck systems", hospital financing consists of global budgets negotiated between the associations representing the various insurance funds and those of hospitals.
DRG	System of hospital financing based on hospital admissions, valued for a price list defined on the allocation of each admission to one single DRG (Diagnosis-Related Group).

Country	DRG state and features
Austria: DRGs	Developed, LFK-PCS.
East Europe: DRGs	Adapted, HBCS based on CMS-DRG (Hungary); adapted, JPG based on HRG (Poland).
Finland: DRGs	Adapted, Nord-DRG based on CMS-DRG.
Germany: DRGs	Adapted, G-DRG based on AN-DRG ("Institute for the Hospital Remuneration System" INek). 80% of hospital revenues are based on DRGs; high-cost drugs, devices and procedures are covered by additional funding.
Greece: DRGs	Adopted, G-DRG, trail - MoU with Germany.
Italy: DRGs	Adopted, CMS-DRG (Ministry of Health). Some functions (DEA, File F) have a separate reimbursement.
Netherlands: DRGs	Developed, DBCs system (Diagnosis Treatments Combinations), pricing system similar to DRGs but based on the combination of therapeutic areas. The calculation of DBCs consists of two elements: Segment A, a fixed share is determined at national level, it is estimated on a prospective budget and negotiated with the associations of providers and of insurances; Segment B: directly negotiated between private insurances and hospitals, today this segment weighs 35% in the price-related calculation.
Spain: DRGs	Adopted, AP-DRG based on CMS-DRG in Catalonia.
United States: DRGs	Developed, MS-DRG also AP-DRG and APR-DRG. There are two types of coverage plans to provide services: Fee For Service and Managed Care Organizations.

Hybrid system DRG/Budget	
Country	DRG state and features
Belgium: DRGs	Adopted, APR-DRG; budget.
Denmark/Sweden:	Adapted, Nord-DRG based on CMS-DRG; global budget.
East Europe: DRGs	Adapted, SL-DRG based on G-DRG; budget (Slovakia). Adopted, IR-DRG; budget (Czech Republic).
France: DRGs, global budget	Developed, HRG, first version based on CMS-DRG. Public and non-profit hospitals negotiate a general budget at regional level and they are paid on a monthly basis; those for profit are

(cont.) →

Table 20.2 *(continued)*

	reimbursed through negotiated rates with the Government. 56% of hospital revenues are based on DRGs; organ transplants, high-cost drugs, devices, research and emergency care are covered by additional funding.
Ireland: DRGs	Adopted, AR-DRG; global budget.
Portugal: DRGs	Adopted, AP-DRG; global budget.
United Kingdom: DRGs (previously budget)	Developed, HRG ("Health and Social Care Information Centre-National Casemix Office"). The system of "Payment by results" was introduced for the reimbursement of hospital care that determines variability of the refunded fee and of the use of the Health Resource Group pricing system (a variation of the DRGs). 60% of hospital revenues are based on DRGs; high-cost drugs, devices and procedures are covered by additional funding.

Table 20.3 Discharges for abdominal wall surgery DRGs 159, 160, 161, 162, 163 in the first half of 2015 in Italy

Region	DRG 159	DRG 160	DRG 161	DRG 162	DRG 163	Total
Piemonte	120	1182	168	4100	95	5665
Lombardia	215	2167	283	4063	256	6984
Valle d'Aosta	4	12	25	60	1	102
P.A. Bolzano	9	53	21	81	22	186
P.A. Trento	4	59	16	74	1	154
Veneto	115	793	127	712	84	1831
Friuli Venezia G.	38	285	65	567	23	978
Liguria	53	213	84	264	10	624
Emilia-Romagna	111	1195	213	2387	272	4178
Toscana	131	810	237	1544	55	2777
Umbria	26	252	58	862	35	1233
Marche	44	397	75	1306	42	1864
Lazio	154	1063	206	1896	183	3502
Abruzzo	45	253	75	612	46	1031
Molise	10	54	26	96	2	188
Campania	117	879	234	2263	119	3612
Puglia	154	690	347	1995	324	3510
Basilicata	18	119	56	351	27	571
Calabria	22	164	80	351	54	671
Sicilia	101	613	175	778	116	1783
Sardegna	51	321	87	899	59	1417

Source: http://www.salute.gov.it/portale/documentazione/p6_2_8_3_1.jsp?lingua=italiano&id=24

as open hernioplasty with suture or prosthesis, posterior or anterior prosthetic open approach, laparoscopic or robotic technologies. The use of any of these techniques entails a different drain on resources in terms of operating theatre utilization, medical devices, number of professionals involved. Furthermore, even if the same open procedure were performed in each case, patients could still differ in clinical homeostasis, requiring an unequal expenditure of resources because of pre-surgery consultations and examinations or post-surgery follow-up visits (patients on oral anticoagulation therapy).

Finally, even in the absence of the three mentioned biases – use of medical devices, resources for pre-surgery or post-surgery assistance – patients may have hernias of different size from PL1M0F0 to giant inguinoscrotal hernia, multirecurrent R2L3M2F0 hernia, even though analysis of a large database does not seem to indicate that size affects mean or median theatre occupation time. As regards the health economics analysis of the five-year database of the ASST Grande Ospedale Metropolitano Niguarda involving 3,470 cases of abdominal wall hernia in adult patients, this shows that surgical time in unilateral hernioplasty (1,984 cases) is related to competence and complexity of the case. Consultants with a high volume of operations have better performance (Figs. 20.1 and 20.2).

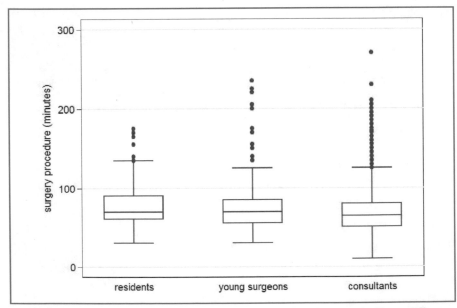

Fig. 20.1 Competence-age of surgeon. The one-way ANOVA shows a significant difference between time duration for consultants and for residents, in the sense that surgeries performed by consultants have lower duration (F test: $p=0.0011$; Scheffé test: $p=0.003$). No significant differences were found between young surgeons and residents or young surgeons and consultants (Scheffé test: $p=0.061$, and $p>0.999$, respectively). The same result is also confirmed by the Kruskal-Wallis test ($p<0.0001$). The Jonckheere-Terpstra test for trend ($p<0.0001$) shows that time duration between classes has a significantly linear trend

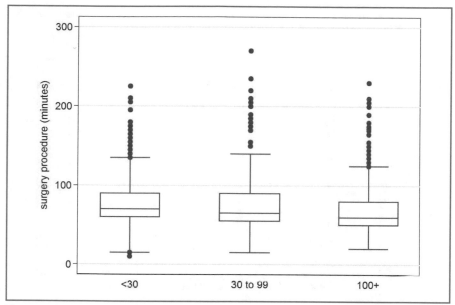

Fig. 20.2 Competence-number of hernioplasties performed over 5 years. The one-way ANOVA shows a significant difference between time duration for surgeons with 100+ operations and surgeons with fewer operations, in the sense that surgeries performed by those with a higher number of operations last less (F test: $p<0.0001$; Scheffé test: $p<0.001$ for comparison 100+ vs. 30-99; $p<0.001$ for comparison 100+ vs. <30; $p>0.999$ for comparison between 30 to 99 vs.<30). The same result is confirmed also by the Kruskal-Wallis test ($p<0.0001$). The Jonckheere-Terpstra test for trend ($p<0.0001$) shows that time duration between classes has a significantly linear trend

Day surgery hernioplasty absorbs fewer resources in terms of surgical time than inpatient or urgency cases (Fig. 20.3).

Hernioplasty DRG 161, 162, 163 may be provided as a "day hospital"[1] procedure. DRG 162 has 63.0% of cases provided in outpatients, with a variation from 12.3% (Calabria region) to 90.8 % (Piemonte region) according to the organization of the different regional healthcare systems (Fig. 20.4).

20.3.   Drain on Resources

20.3.1 Hospital Resources

Performance of a surgical procedure [14] requires clinical, nursing or administrative resources in addition to theatre resources, the indicator of which is turnover time [15]. We identify these resources through a specific pathway defined "surgical path-

---

[1] *Ordinary admission*: hospitalization for 2 and 7 days. *Day hospital*: hospitalization for 1 day, with an overnight stay in some regions.

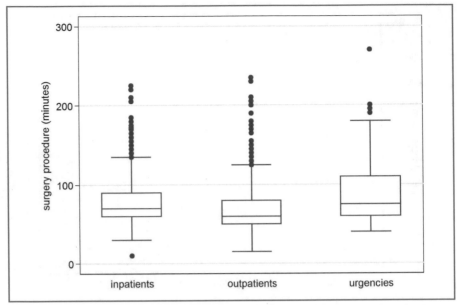

Fig. 20.3 Complexity of the cases. The one-way ANOVA shows a significant difference between time duration depending on the patient's hospital status, in the sense that surgeries performed in outpatients last less than surgeries in inpatients and in urgencies (F test: p<0.0001; Scheffé test: p<0.001 for comparison inpatients vs. outpatients; p<0.001 for comparison inpatients vs. urgencies; p<0.001 for comparison outpatients vs. urgencies). The same result is confirmed also by the Kruskal-Wallis test (p<0.0001). The Jonckheere-Terpstra test for trend (p=0.0132) shows that time duration between classes has a significantly linear trend

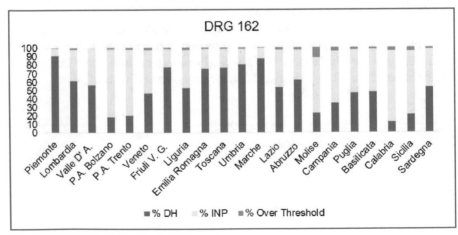

Fig. 20.4 DRG 162 distribution in Italian regions

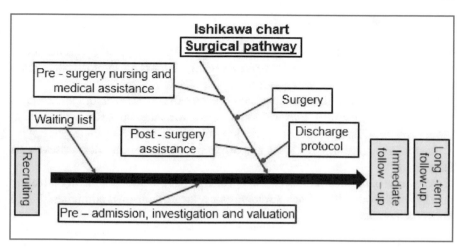

Fig. 20.5 Ishikawa flow chart

way" [15, 16]. This includes a combination of phases from outpatient recruiting to the patient's discharge from the same pathway, after the early follow-up.

The pathway can be illustrated by means of a number of different flow charts, though we prefer an Ishikawa [17, 18] chart (Fig. 20.5) that splits a process into steps, giving everyone a function in order to identify human, logistic, clinical, and nursing resources used. We can identify at each level the number of professionals involved and the standard time or we can identify how many procedures each professional can produce yearly. Afterwards we can estimate the overall cost of the single part of the procedure. An example could be the management of the waiting list. The administrative division is involved (one administrative clerk can handle an average of 1,500 cases) in scheduling (prehospital admission, surgery, follow-up), management of clinical documentation etc., plus overhead costs[2].

The same analysis can be performed on prehospital admission [19]. The amount of resources consumed depends on the type of procedure and illness class of the patient, and associated diseases. Inguinal hernioplasty, performed as day surgery in more than half of the cases, includes only preanesthetic evaluation for ASA 1-2 patients <60 years of age, a pool of blood tests [glycemia, creatinine, complete blood count (CBC), PT (prothrombin time), PTT (activated partial thromboplastin time)], ECG, chest X-ray and preanesthetic evaluation for those >60 years, whereas further investigations for associated diseases such as diabetes, cardiovascular or neurological diseases may be necessary for ASA 3 patients.

---

[2] Overhead cost is 30% of the total cost.

20.3.2   Medical Devices

Specific devices: hernia mesh. This depends on both the type of intervention and the cost of the mesh that may vary from few cents [20, 21] mosquito mesh to more than 100 euros or dollars for laparoscopic intervention.

Generic devices: this includes disposable or reusable nonwoven drapes, sutures, electric scalpel, surgical gloves, green coats for surgical team and patient, monitoring tools, surgical set amortization, anesthetic set.

Drugs: anesthetic drugs for local or peripheral blocks, antibiotics, intravenous feeding.

General cost of the theatre: this is strictly related to the single hospital organization and has wide variability. Each surgeon can refer to their own administration to know the precise cost.

20.3.3   Staff Costs

Theatre: it is necessary to change approach and calculate staff time based not on surgical time [22–25] but on turnover time[3], which is surgical time plus anesthesiology time, sanification input and discharge of the patient. From the perspective of costs, it can be concluded that the average operating theatre utilization is estimated to be 100' for unilateral inguinal hernia procedures done with local anesthesia and 120' for procedures done with general anesthesia; as for bilateral inguinal hernia, theatre utilization amounts to 127' and 157', respectively [25]. We have to evaluate the number of professionals involved so the time becomes:

* surgeon time 5.25 h
* anesthesiologist 1 1.20 h
* nursing time: each operating block needs two nurses and one nursing assistant who are able to provide 800 unilateral inguinal hernia procedures over one year.

Our data show a mean time for open unilateral inguinal repair of 71.7 min and a median of 65 min; for a VDL procedure the mean is 96.4 and the median is 90. Turnover time becomes 120 min for open hernioplasty and 140 min for VDL procedures.

Nursing costs: day surgery bed cost. This is calculated by dividing the number of beds multiplied the number of days of activity by the number of nurses multiplied by their annual salary. In our setting, a day surgery bed costs 57.32 euro. For inpatients, beds cost 100 euro daily.

---

[3] From the time one patient leaves the room until the next patient enters, including preparation and discharge time as well as anesthesiology, clinical and disinfecting time.

20.4   Costs Involved

The involved costs included in the analysis are:
- loss of productivity of patients in waiting list
  - working days lost by patients in waiting list
- loss of quality life for seniors

Currently, there is no EBM pricing for this type of costs or for the fairness of access to care.

20.5   Conclusions

Currently, Italy uses the DRG reimbursement system, the fees of which are shown in Fig. 20.6. The fees cover costs for an outpatient open procedure for a primary unilateral hernia but not for bilateral or recurrent hernias, particularly if done in VDL with general anesthesia.

We can conclude with a Level 1B recommendation from the European Hernia Society guidelines [26]: "From the perspective of the hospital, an open mesh procedure is the most cost-effective operation in primary unilateral hernias. From a socio-economic perspective, an endoscopic procedure is probably the most cost-effective approach for patients who participate in the labour market, especially for bilateral hernias".

So, in this first phase, it could be concluded that the inhomogeneity of the cluster, caused by the dispersion of the cases within it, affects the use of resources

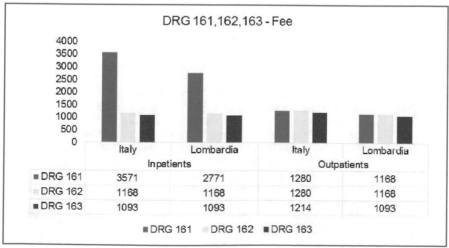

Fig. 20.6 Fees in the Lombardia region and fees for exchange between regions

so that a reimbursement of this type (a single tariff rate) is not equitable for this group of diseases, even though our experience shows a total cost that is less than in the current literature [25].

References

1. Saita M (1996) Programmazione e controllo. Centro studi aziendali. Giuffrè, Milano
2. Brailer DJ (1998) Clinical performance improvement: measuring costs and benefits. Med Prat Manage 14:31–34
3. Berger K, Szucs TD (1999) Socioeconomic evaluation in medicine in Europe. Core economic concepts. Pharmaeconomics 16 (Suppl 1):19–25
4. Shafer W, Kroneman M, Boerma W et al (2010) Health Systems in Transition: The Netherlands. European Observatory on Systems and Polices. http://www.euro.who.int/data/assets/pdf_file/0008/85391/E93667.pdf
5. Chevreul K Durand-Zaleski I, Bahrami SB et al (2010) France: Health system review. Health Systems in Transition. European Health Observatory Study Series
6. Zarlino EJ, Piontek FA, Kohli R (1999) The utility of hospital administrative data for gene rating a screening program to predict adverse outcomes. Am J Med Qual 14:242–247
7. Nicholson D (2010) Liberating the NHS: managing the transition. Department of Health www.dh.gov.uk/prod_consum_dh/groups/dh_digitalassets/documents/digitalasset/dh_117406.pdf
8. Bellini I (2014) Il Sistema Sanitario Tedesco. Salute Internazionale Info. http://www.saluteinternazionale.info/2014/09/il-sistema-sanitario-tedesco/
9. Ministero della Salute (2013) Finanziamento del SSN. http://www.salute.gov.it/portale/salute/p1_5.jsp?id=66&area=Il_Ssn
10. Fattore G (2010) I modelli e la storia dei sistemi sanitari in Europa e Stati Uniti. In: Zangrandi A (ed) Economia e management per le professioni sanitarie. McGraw Hill, Milano, pp 63–78
11. Veneziano MA, Specchia ML (2010) Il sistema sanitario spagnolo. Salute Internazionale Info. http://www.saluteinternazionale.info/2010/12/il-sistema-sanitario-spagnolo/
12. Centers for Medicare and Medicaid Services https://www.cms.gov/
13. Lorenzoni L (2015) Il sistema di finanziamento dell'attività degli ospedali basato sui DRG: il contesto internazionale. IT-DRG meeting, Rome 11 March 2015 drgit.agenas.it/Handlers/dochandler.ashx?id=36
14. Nicosia F (2010) Il nuovo ospedale è snello. Far funzionare gli ospedali con il Lean Healthcare: consigli pratici e sostenibilità. Franco Angeli, Milano
15. Buccioli M, Grementieri P, Signani R et al (2012) Qualità e sicurezza del paziente chirurgico: information technology per la governance di un percorso integrato. Evidence 4(1)
16. Garner P (2012) Complexities in the operating room. In: Lim G, Herrmann JW (eds) Proceedings of the 2012 Industrial and Systems Engineering Research Conference
17. Greco DP (2000) Dal protocollo alla tariffa: un percorso per affrontare e gestire le problematiche dei costi della sanità. Franco Angeli, Milano
18. Ishikawa K (1997) Guida al controllo di qualità. Franco Angeli, Milano
19. Sandberg WS, Daily B, Egan M et al (2005) Deliberate perioperative systems design improves operating room throughput. Anesthesiology 103:406–418
20. Yang J, Papandria D, Rhee Det al (2011) Low-cost mesh for inguinal hernia repair in resource-limited settings. Hernia 15:485–489
21. Löfgren J, Nordin P, Ibingira C et al (2016) A randomized trial of low-cost mesh in groin hernia repair. N Engl J Med 374:146–153
22. Weinbroum AA, Ekstein P, Ezri T (2003) Efficiency of the operating room suite. Am J Surg 185:244–250

23. Surgery Management Improvement Group (2012) Rapid Operating Room Turnover. http://
     www.surgerymanagement.com/presentations/rapid-operating-room-turnover1.php
24. Cendàn JC, Good M (2006) Interdisciplinary work flow assessment and redesign decreases
     operating room turnover time and allows for additional caseload. Arch Surg 141:65–69
25. Tadaki C, Lomelin D, Simorov A et al (2016) Perioperative outcomes and costs of
     laparoscopic versus open inguinal hernia repair. Hernia [Epub ahead of print] doi:10.1007/
     s10029-016-1465-y
26. Simons MP, Aufenacker T, Bay-Nielsen M et al (2009) European Hernia Society guidelines
     on the treatment of inguinal hernia in adult patients. Hernia 13:343–403

Printed in the United States
By Bookmasters